THE FACT[...]

D[...]

- Even a back attack tha[...] need not become a chronic n[...]

- Stress alone is *not* the cause of your backache. While psychological factors can complicate your pain, your back hurts because something has happened to it.

- Excess weight increases the chances of recurring back trouble.

- Good posture is essential. A heavy bag carried over the shoulder tends to result in uneven shoulders and puts stress on the back muscles.

Give your back the treatment it deserves! Everything you need to know can be found in . . .

RELIEF FROM CHRONIC BACKACHE

THE DELL MEDICAL LIBRARY

THE DELL MEDICAL LIBRARY

Relief from
CHRONIC
BACKACHE

Edmund Blair Bolles

Foreword by Jackson Tan, M.D., P.T.

A LYNN SONBERG BOOK

Correct diagnosis of the cause of pain and the proper course of treatment are matters that require individual attention from a physician. In addition, back pain can be a symptom of illnesses (such as kidney disease) that do not involve the muscles and other tissues of the back and that would not respond to the methods described in this book. Any person who suffers back pain should therefore consult a physician before beginning the exercises described in this book or any other course of treatment. The reader should bear in mind that this book is not for the purpose of self-diagnosis or self-treatment and that any and all medical problems should be referred to the expertise of appropriate medical personnel.

Published by
Dell Publishing
a division of
Bantam Doubleday Dell Publishing Group, Inc.
666 Fifth Avenue
New York, New York 10103

Published by arrangement with Lynn Sonberg Book Services, 166 East 56 Street, New York, New York 10022.

ISBN: 0-440-20571-9

Printed in the United States of America
Published simultaneously in Canada
June 1990

10 9 8 7 6 5

OPM

CONTENTS

ACKNOWLEDGMENTS

I wish to thank the following medical experts for their generosity in taking the time to answer my questions and sharing their expertise:

Dr. Isaac Pinter, director of the Orthopaedic-Arthritis Pain Center, the Hospital for Joint Diseases Orthopaedic Institute in New York City

Dr. Willibald Nagler, physiatrist-in-chief, New York Hospital–The Cornell Medical Center

Dr. Edythe M. Heus, applied kinesiologist, Union Square Chiropractic

and

Jackson Tan, M.D., senior physical therapist of the Pain Center at the Hospital for Joint Diseases

FOREWORD

Low-back pain is a common costly problem affecting an estimated 50 to 80 percent of America's working population at least once during their career. Many people, of course, are affected more than once and some people find that the pain becomes a continuing part of their lives. Besides the damage done to individuals, back pain is expensive. In terms of medical care and lost workdays it costs billions of dollars every year.

We at the Pain Center see the great range of people affected directly and indirectly by back pain. Family members, employers, insurance companies, and lawyers are involved as well as the patient. We also see the way back pain can make emotions run high. The majority of low-back pains are due to mechanical injuries—strains and sprains—to the soft tissue (i.e., muscles or ligaments of the spine), and these problems do not show up on the objective tests available to medicine. The images produced by X rays, myelograms, CAT scans, or MRI do not reveal these injuries even though the patient can feel them intensely.

The conflict between the patient's misery and the inability of testing to explain the suffering has the potential of becoming more entangled. The patient who is also an employee may want workmen's compensation, which the employer, in the absence of definitive diagnosis, is reluctant to pay. Some of the patients we see become involved in lawsuits with employers who charge them with malingering. Although the employer's complaint is sometimes justified, studies have shown that the majority of patients are bona fide back-pain sufferers. Instead of trying to take advantage of the confusion brought on by soft-tissue damage, they are its legal as well as physical victims.

The treatment of low-back pain has always focused on the alleviation of the pain without much emphasis on its accompanying functional impairments. Such impairments include psychological, social, and physical damage. Each day at the Pain Center we see how much more there is to treating back pain than the bed rest and narcotic pain medications that are usually prescribed by physicians who hope to control the pain. Back surgery is performed excessively, even though its long-term success in pain reduction is very low. We see the results of these partial approaches: "chronic pain" patients who are dependent on pain medications, physically out of condition, mentally depressed, and socially withdrawn.

The majority of chronic-pain patients I see at the Pain Center of the Hospital for Joint Diseases Orthopaedic Institute are low-back-pain sufferers. Most of them need narcotic painkillers just to do their daily activities and are out of shape physically, psychologically, and socially. Financially, too, they are in bad shape, and most of them have pending lawsuits or workman's compensation claims. The majority also have had previous back surgery and have received some form of passive treatment such as the use of hot packs, ultrasound, spinal manipulation, traction, and so forth. Active exercises, like the ones described in this book, were usually excluded from their treatment plan since most physicians *do not* prescribe them. Even if the patients had been given physical exercises by their physical therapists, the majority of them did not comply since they were specifically told by their doctors not to exercise when in pain. Most strikingly, many of the patients that I encounter are totally ignorant about their backs despite having undergone multiple back surgeries!

It is unfortunate that our health-care system emphasizes "treatment" instead of "prevention" of diseases. If we had put more resources into public health education and preventive medicine, telling, for example, back-pain sufferers the facts provided in this book, the current financial crisis of our health-care systems might have been avoided. I strongly believe that the majority of low-back-pain patients could have been prevented from becoming chronic sufferers—if only the health professionals they turned to had focused less on surgery, medications, and/or relying on passive treatments and had spent more time educating their patients about the active care of their backs as well as the importance of restoring physical function after an episode of back pain.

Concise and informative books such as this one play a vital role in the solution to the complex problem of low-back pain. Mr. Bolles describes an active treatment program. It does not ignore surgery, prescription medications, and passive treatment, but it places the emphasis where it should be—on active care and the restoration of physical function. The book seeks not only to educate readers about their backs but also to let them participate in the treatment of their back problems. Hopefully, it will decrease both the physical and mental anguish of readers as well as help them to avoid the social and economic disasters I have seen low-back pain bring.

—JACKSON TAN, M.D., P.T.,
*Orthopaedic-Arthritis Pain
Center, Hospital for Joint
Diseases Orthopaedic Institute*

INTRODUCTION:
A NEW LOOK AT AN
OLD PROBLEM

"Biology has its surprises," said a world-renowned back-ache expert over lunch. He was considering the changes that have come during his career of relieving back pain. He explained his point about surprises: Doctors used to think that the human back should be a certain way. It should be as straight as possible (excepting a slight curve in the lumbar, or lower, area). It should not move too much. It should not have too many knobs and bumps on it. Whenever doctors examined the spines of backache patients the X rays and a special kind of image known as a myelogram revealed all sorts of spinal "abnormalities." The doctors assumed that there, in those idiosyncrasies, lay the problem. The result was an aggressive program of surgery to reshape a patient's back. Sometimes it helped dramatically, but *more often* surgery was unnecessary. Eventually doctors began to ask why these supposed abnormalities were also present in the X rays of people who had never had a backache. The old theorizers had forgotten about biology's variability. Living things are not standardized. Recent research has astonished the traditionalists by showing there is no meaningful relationship between the old standards and a person's backache. The familiar

1

wisdom about sitting and standing straight, wisdom we all grew up with, does not apply. Advice about posture was not really nonsense, but it offered no useful guidance about what to do once your back begins to hurt.

This book tells you what to do—what to do when your back hurts and how to avoid the recurrence of pain. It takes into account the many surprises medicine has faced during the past decades. Included are the following, none of which could have appeared had this book been written in the mid-1970s:

• Your backache does not have to become chronic. The old belief to the contrary is outdated. Medicine has discovered new ways of responding to back pain. Even a back attack that twists you like a pretzel and sends you to bed for a week should never become a chronic misery.

• You can exercise to restore back function. This book does more than offer a variety of exercises to help get bad backs into shape. It also tells you when particular exercises are appropriate and how to judge your performance. Backache can almost always be treated successfully if a sufferer can get comfortable enough to engage in a rehabilitative exercise program. In the past backache exercises were offered as a way to try warding off future troubles. That approach was not terribly successful; people did their exercises and still injured their backs. The point of the exercises in this book is *rehabilitation*.

• Medicine's attitude toward back pain has changed. It has become more tolerant of the idiosyncrasies of patients. Proper posture helps, of course, and there are other ideals as well, but few of us can live up to them all. Medicine has grown more forgiving. No longer do doctors shrug and say it is your own fault when your back begins to hurt. Readers will find a chapter on how to avoid problems in the future, but even though you may not have lived up to the ideals, you can still find a path to full recovery.

The surprises of the last dozen years have brought much more hope than once seemed possible. Even if this book had been written as recently as the mid-1980s, it could not have been as practical and encouraging as it is. As medicine began to realize that individual variation did not explain backache, some doctors began to say the whole problem was in the patient's head. Psychological tension was cited as *the* source of backache. Fortunately, that phase of medical theory was short-lived. You will find much discussion of stress, both physical and emotional, in this book, but stress alone is not the cause of your backache. Psychological factors can complicate your pain, but back pain has physical origins. The good news reported in these pages is just that simple: Your back hurts because something happened to it. It can get better if you know what to do. This book will tell you what you need to know.

Medicine has learned what people can do about their backaches, which allows this book to take on a new organization. In the past, books about backache began with chapters that discussed the anatomy of the back in rich detail and then they surveyed all the many rare diseases of the spine. They read like medical texts written for lay people. Practical discussion of exercises and anything else the author cared to recommend was usually left to the final few chapters. This book is organized in precisely the opposite way. Practical information comes first. The details of anatomy and rare disease have been left for the back of the book. Readers who care to learn more can look there, but first of all this book offers a practical application of today's medicine.

The first two chapters explain what has gone wrong in the majority of back problems and introduce a practical program that will let you reclaim your full life.

The bulk of the book looks at what readers need to do at a particular stage of their back pain. Back attacks go through a regular series of phases, starting with *acute backache*. Chapter 3 takes you through that painful time, telling you what to do day by day. Acute backache is a relatively brief stage that turns into a longer *recovery period*. Chapter 4 explores this second stage of backache and is similar to the acute backache chapter in the way it offers practical what-to-do information. Chapter 5 then discusses the *after-backache* stage. One hopes that this stage will continue for the rest of a former sufferer's life. Like other chapters, this one includes practical information about what to do to stay healthy and how to respond if your back begins to warn of recurring trouble.

Each of these chapters closes with a discussion of which backache practitioners may be of help at each stage of a back attack. Many readers will find that they do not need to consult a professional, but if you feel that you do need help, you will soon learn that there is a bewildering array of specialists in treating backache. Should you see a doctor or a chiropractor? What about acupuncturists and hypnotists? Do multidiscipline approaches help? The answers to these questions depend on what stage of a back attack you are experiencing. Acute attack calls for one type of specialist, recovery another. And if you are in chronic pain, you may need someone different again. There are also specialists who are good for after the back attack. It is important to see the right practitioner at the right stage. Most backache victims find that their friends have many stories to tell. Some had great success with a chiropractor, others say just the opposite. Some liked their orthopedist, others hated theirs. Besides individual differences, these contradictions probably reflect the stage at which a person encountered a particular practitioner. Get one at the right stage and miracles seem to follow. Get the same professional at the wrong stage and disappointment results.

The final chapters of the book offer information for people who need, or want, to know more. The first is about chronic backache, pain that does not go away, even after months or years. The earlier chapters were designed explicitly to help readers avoid surgery or suffering chronic pain, but some people will already be in the chronic-pain stage when they pick up this book. They need to know that their problem can be treated. The chapter on chronic pain discusses how to reduce its presence and get back on the road to recovery.

Chapter 7 is about surgery. Much too much back surgery is done, but sometimes it *is* necessary. This chapter will help you make an informal decision. Finally, there is a "ready reference," a glossary of terms that readers may encounter as they endure their backache. This contains the description of back vertebrae and ligaments. It also provides a quick reference to terms used in the earlier chapters.

As a person who has suffered some severe back attacks myself, researching the information for this book was both encouraging and rewarding. Like millions of others, I had my fears of recurrence and I obeyed my superstitions about how to avoid another bout, but I had no clear notion of what to do when pain actually struck. If I bent over to pick up a crying child, or stood up from a hard day at the keyboard and felt my back let out a shriek, I knew plenty of fear but nothing that was practical. I am grateful to the many researchers in this field whose writings showed me what was happening. I also appreciate the help of other backache sufferers who spoke freely about their experiences. I must also thank the practicing experts who gladly told me what they have learned. In particular I want to thank Dr. Isaac Pinter, the director of the Orthopaedic-Arthritis Pain Center, the Hospital for Joint Diseases Orthopaedic Institute in New York City; Dr. Willibald Nagler, physiatrist-in-chief, New York Hospital—The Cornell Medical Center; Dr. Edythe M. Heus, applied kinesiologist, Union Square Chiropractic; and Dr. Jackson C. Tan, senior physical therapist of the Pain Center at the Hospital for Joint Diseases. Each of these specialists generously took the time to answer my questions and show me what I

needed to know to bring this book right up to date.
Jackson Tan even took the trouble of reading the entire
manuscript and making suggestions. Any remaining er-
rors are my fault, but I thank him for his thoughtful
guidance.

E.B.B.

RECLAIMING
YOUR LIFE

Backache cannot kill you, but sufferers do know a special kind of fear. They worry that they will hurt this way for the rest of their life. A first back attack commonly strikes people between age twenty-five and thirty-five. Several studies have even found that nearly one fifth (18 percent) of women and men twenty-four years old and younger have already had their first back problem. These people have their whole lives ahead of them when a sudden biting ache raises the question of what kind of life the long decades will be. First-time sufferers may not have paid much attention before to references to lumbago, slipped disks, and "Oh, my aching back," but now memories of those remarks rise up like ghosts to haunt the imagination. The sufferer asks, "Didn't Uncle Joe have to take early retirement because of a bad back? And I am half his age!" A vision of a life in pain terrifies the spirit.

At stake are sufferers' view of themselves as friends, adults, parents, lovers, and active doers. Pain attacks the body but strips away the pleasures of the soul as well. Doctors may point out that less than 4 percent of back-ache sufferers find their lives filled with persistent pain bouts. At a time like this, however, statistics are no comfort. Patients want to know that they are not going to be in that tiny minority.

People who have had back pains before may feel less panicky at the first flare-up of a new attack. They know these pangs come from time to time and they have found some ritual, like sleeping on the floor for three consecutive nights, to overcome the problem. But if the ritual does not work, or if the problem is more than a twinge, then they experience fear for the everyday *pleasures* of their lives.

"Pleasure" may seem like an alien word to back pain sufferers. As a former (knock wood) sufferer myself, I know the immobilizing, astonishing pain that can come from a damaged back. Like millions of other people, I learned I had a bad back in one sudden, sharp, paralyzing moment. I was a graduate student, just turning twenty-four, taking a final exam. I reached for some more writing paper and *zot,* it was as though a werewolf had bitten my back and would not let go. I half stood, bent and frozen, my arm outstretched and unmoving. With the professor leaning forward in old-man style, and me stuck still, the passing of the paper was one of the most difficult physical contests of my entire twenty years of schooling. In truth, a race between a seventy-year-old and a person suffering an acute attack of back agony is no contest. He handed me the paper and I fell back into my seat. *So that is pain.* If anybody had spoken to me about pleasure just then, I would have thought him insane. I did not care about pleasure. I just never wanted to have such pain again.

My attitude, however, was one of the symptoms of serious backache. Sufferers begin to think in terms of a smaller life—one they can cope with, one without pain, or at least one with manageable pain. People who have never suffered from chronic pain can hardly imagine such an attitude. They are mostly familiar with acute pain, those sudden grasping warnings that something is wrong. Acute pain is unwelcome, but often useful. It alerts us to the need to save ourselves and motivates a person to try to restore things to normal. Chronic pain, however, serves no useful function. It only wears us down, drains away ambition, and makes us dread the thought of more pain. In the worst cases it steals so much ambition that just getting through the day begins to seem like a major achievement.

The first job of a backache sufferer, therefore, is to hang on to ambition and insist on reclaiming a full life. Over five million Americans are estimated to suffer serious back problems each year. The number with twinges and pangs is many times higher. Chronic backache is the number one reason people miss working days and is a prime reason for early retirement in every industrial country. It may permanently disable as many as a quarter of a million Americans each year. Back pain has been with humanity for thousands of years, but today it has risen to the level of a plague. The more economically and industrially advanced a country is, the more likely it seems to suffer from an epidemic of back pain. Backache cuts short the working lives of employees in Japan, Sweden, England, and throughout the developed world. Communist countries like Czechoslovakia report that it is a major source of worker disability.

Because of its important economic consequences, industries and governments around the world have scrambled to learn more. Their money has financed new discoveries about an ancient problem. Recent years have also brought important insights into the nature of pain. Pain is one of medicine's deepest mysteries as well as one of humanity's most basic experiences. Relentless backache raises the puzzle of why pain persists when, for all that a doctor can see, the physical trauma was healed long ago. This book uses the latest research and clinical experience to answer one question: What can backache sufferers do to reclaim their full lives as quickly as possible?

The book does not devote much space to the question of assigning blame for the original problem. Many people blame themselves, but it is not your fault that your back hurts. Most of us think it is. We stand up, pain grabs us by surprise, and we say to ourselves, "I must have been sitting wrong." Or after a long peace, pain suddenly returns, and a doctor says, "You weren't doing your exercises." A would-be comforter says, "I told you to see my chiropractor." All of these voices have one message in common: You did something wrong, and now you must pay. This attitude is almost always wrong.

Other people blame the back itself. Folk wisdom, sometimes coming from doctors, holds that the back did not adapt well to the demands of walking on two legs instead of four. Maybe thirty years ago that idea made some sense; biologists still thought upright walking was a recent development. Investigators have since found fossil backbones and footprints, however, that show our ancestors have been walking upright for millions of years. It is one of our oldest human traits, and our bodies have innumerable adaptations to handle the demands of upright walking. Given half a chance, the human back can overcome immense abuse.

A third candidate for blame is the sufferer's employer. Occupational risks to the back come from jobs that demand heavy lifting, or surround a worker with persistent vibration, or require prolonged sitting. In other words most jobs today place the back at risk. Employees should be alert to conditions that can reduce the risk of further back trouble, and this book will provide guidelines in that area, but brooding over blame—whether it be blame for yourself, your boss, or your anatomy—interferes with recovery. In the worst cases it can even block recovery. This fact may seem farfetched. What can something as subjective as attitude have to do with something as real as the back? The answer is plenty. Attitude seldom brings on a back attack, but it is important in recovery.

HOW STRESS HURTS
YOUR BACK

At the outset of a back attack doctors cannot tell from examining the back which patients are the most likely candidates for prolonged unrelenting back pain. A better clue comes from examining the life and attitude of the patient. There is no relation between personality and getting back pain, but some psychological conditions are associated with a risk for chronic back pain. These include anxiety, depression, hypochondria, and work dissatisfaction. Each of these conditions warn of *unrelieved* emotional stress.

Stress is not a purely negative experience—it keeps our muscles fit and minds alert. It helps our backs stay flexible. Stress can also temporarily relieve or block pain, but unending stress erodes both body and soul. Persistent stress in a backache sufferer can delay or even block recovery, turning the discomfort of a few weeks into months or years of misery. Part of recovering from a back attack means learning how to relax your muscles.

Be careful about understanding what I say about emotional stress. Backache is *not* a psychological problem. Something real has happened. Usually the damage is subtle and beyond the discovery of X rays or other technologies. Recovery from any backache must include a physical program to restore the health of the back. Stress is a part of each person's life, and a healthy back should be able to withstand it. Yet a growing body of medical opinion agrees that stress is a major component of backache and is probably the most important factor in delaying recovery.

Stress takes many forms. Physically it includes a tightening of the muscles and a release of various chemicals into the bloodstream and the brain. The human back is rich in muscles and ligaments that wrap around the bones of the spine or attach to them. They can be overtaxed. Athletes who exercise too energetically without first doing warm-up stretches can stress their backs. Out-of-shape people stress their backs too. Weakened muscles of the upper body and neck increase the stress on the lower-back muscles. Weak stomach muscles also stress the back. Obesity is an especially common source of trouble, for, by extending the stomach muscles, it weakens them. People with arthritis or some other problem that limits their mobility can develop muscular imbalances that stress the back.

The relation between stress and pain depends on circumstances. Stress can put antipain chemicals into the body's system, thus reducing a feeling of pain. For example, a person with a back twinge that slows him down may suddenly move quickly to step out of the way of an oncoming car. The physical responses to stress help in that situation. But stress also tenses the muscles, and muscles that stay tense are subject to strains and sprains.

By itself occasional physical stress should not lead to problems. The back was built to handle many muscular stresses and, once the cause of tension passes, the back should continue functioning well. If a muscle is stressed too much or too long, however, it can make a knot, and knotted muscles put your back at risk. If a person with taut muscles suddenly moves in a new way, the muscles may not adapt in time. Ordinary movements become the final straw toward back pain. Standing up from a chair, clapping in excitement after winning a tense game, bending to pick up something you have just dropped, sneezing, or tying one's shoes can do the damage. There is seldom any cause to look for something special about the way you moved. The problem was in the stressed back muscles, not in the motion.

Stress is the common factor that runs through the stages of backache. Most of the exercises and practices described in this book are for a specific stage of back suffering and are presented in the chapters about the relevant stages. But you should make a specific effort to relax your muscles during the whole period of the back attack. That does not mean you should avoid stress but let the stress pass. Do not keep your muscles taut. Two physical habits to practice during any time of backache problem are:

- *Drink plenty of water.* Eight glasses of water each day help dissolve and eliminate the buildup of stress chemicals. You don't like plain water? Drink it anyway.

- *Shrug your shoulders.* This activity releases tension in the muscles. After an emotional event take a deep breath, pulling your shoulders up with an exaggerated motion as you inhale. Then let them fall, continuing to exhale after the shoulders are down. It relaxes the muscles after emotions have tightened them.

Shoulder shrugging points out the close relation between physical and emotional stress. This physical action is a response to an emotional event. Mastering emotional stress is an important part of your back's physical recovery. Two other practices you should maintain throughout a backache period seek to reduce your psychological stress:

- *Visualization.* Twice each day lie on something sturdy—a bed or the floor—and imagine joyous things for fifteen minutes. Think of places and things that please you. If you are not much at conjuring up images, use words to describe something. (Usually people who turn to words realize they do think in images after all.) If words fail you, recall music. Keep these times happy, and do not think about your back. Do NOT imagine what it will be like when your back is better. Do NOT imagine how your back is getting better. Think of happy times in your life and picture them.

- *Diary.* Keep a detailed record of your day's activities. Mark it daily during the acute stage of the problem, and then weekly during the recovery period. At first this record may be something of a shock as you see exactly how much of your life has been curtailed by your back pain, but as time passes you can see how well you are reclaiming those limits and your life.

STRESS AND PAIN BEHAVIOR

Because of its psychological aspects, stress in backache can become circular. Your back begins to hurt because of damage wrought under tension. And your back muscles are tense now because you are stressed by a hurting back. This cycle can lead to "pain behavior," a term used for a common pattern of behavioral changes in response to chronic pain. Its chief characteristics are declining social responsibility and a growing obsession with avoiding any further hurt. It is because of pain behavior that some thoughtless observers dismiss chronic backache as being "all in the head."

Psychological stress is not easily reduced to one sentence, but its essence combines uncertainty with a need to act. A driver on a highway may suddenly have to swing wide to avoid a collision with another car. That is a stressful moment, full of uncertainty and the need for quick action. Moments like these are a natural part of every life, and when they pass people can relax and even congratulate themselves on having handled a difficult situation well. Such experiences promote self-confidence as the driver thinks, "Driving can be dangerous, but I am up to it."

Now imagine the same incident from the viewpoint of a passenger in the swerving car. The uncertainty is the same. The desire to get out of the way is the same. But the passenger cannot take action. Survival or crash is out of the passenger's control. When the moment passes the passenger may relax again but there is no boost of self-confidence. The passenger, like the driver, has been reminded that riding in a car is dangerous. The passenger thinks, "Driving is dangerous, and I have nothing to do with the outcome." Without that renewed self-confidence, a passenger's response to natural stress is limited to four choices:

• *Become passive:* Docilely accept whatever fate may bring.

• *Grow anxious:* Worry and fuss to no avail.

• *Become depressed:* Glumly await one's own ruin.

• *Deny the problem:* Forget about what just happened.

Back sufferers often feel like a passenger in a swerving car. They have no clear notion of what to do about their pain and feel alienated from their own bodies. In these circumstances many people deny the problem, but that "solution" can last only so long. Eventually those pangs and twinges will grow into an acute attack that forces a person to face the reality of a back problem. Until then the sufferer feels trapped between passivity, anxiety, and depression.

Passivity in the back patient commonly takes the form of reliance on others, notably on doctors or chiropractors. Anyone with chronic back pain should seek help, but even at their best, professionals can only treat the sources of pain. It is up to you to take your life back. When interviewing back sufferers for this book, nothing was more distressing than to see the way some of them passively accepted their shrunken lives, even boasting about it. One man reported:

> I still have occasional pain, but I don't have any more nerve effects. I have had to give up my tennis, because of the twisting motion for serving and for overheads. But I have NOT given up my cross-country skiing— indeed I traveled 168 miles on the snow last winter.

The absent "nerve effects" means the pain is now localized in the back and does not travel into the hips. Yet regularly recurring pain three years after a back attack is not good. This man thinks he has recovered from what he called his "sciatica," and yet tennis has gone out of his life forever. It is true that some studies associate tennis with back risk, but the same research links backache and cross-country skiing as well. Indeed this man's first back attack came when he was cross-country skiing. The difference appears to be that he loves the skiing enough to insist on keeping it in his life. He has let the tennis go and the "docs," as he calls them, encourage him to believe he has recovered. He has made progress. He has returned to work and is functioning. He is not one of those people who swell the numbers of the permanently disabled. But recurring pain is a regular part of his life and his life is less active than it was. Passive acceptance of this fate is not the way to reclaim your life after a back attack.

Anxiety is an even more unfortunate response to back pain. It can trigger a terrible cycle: Anxiety leads to greater pain; the greater pain leads to still greater anxiety, which, of course, produces still more pain. This anxiety cycle can then take on all sorts of bizarre complexities, especially in a person's dealing with others. In the early days of a back attack most sufferers can look forward to sympathy from family and friends, but sympathies wane as time passes. Even doctors will say that a person is exaggerating or imagining the pain. All that pooh-poohing increases the sufferer's anxiety, so the pain and sense of helplessness grow. In the worst cases anxiety can shrink a back sufferer's life to the size of a small bed in a small room.

Depression is another response that contributes to pain. Depressed people tend to be less assertive than anxious people, so a depressed back patient may be less wearisome to others, but otherwise depression can lead to the same behavior seen among anxious people. We see the same cycles of pain feeding on emotions and we see the widespread accusation of malingering. Depression plus backache can lead to a lifetime disability.

The passive search for someone else to save your back, the anxious avoidance of any action that might disturb the back, and the depressed refusal to believe help is possible are all hallmarks of "pain behavior." Doctors see the results routinely in their practice. Whenever backache strikes a person is at some risk of pain behavior. Even if the back recovers and the pain fades, the memory of the pain may still affect behavior, especially if a person does not know what to do. If you know how to take care of your back, you should be able to escape the vicious circle of pain behavior.

AVOIDING PAIN BEHAVIOR

Recovery from backache requires two responses to stress. Since every backache sufferer will, to some extent, experience anxiety, depression, and passivity, each person must individually

- find the strength to overcome these moods and

- avoid dashing right back into a life of persistent stresses.

Most people have plenty of motivation to recover fully: They want to get on with their lives and cannot endure the shrunken existence that comes with chronic backache. Others may not be quite so in love with life, but they have too many obligations to stay in bed. A few patients, however, already had shrunken lives before their backaches started. Their work was an unsatisfying drudgery that they continued only because they needed the income. The need for an income might still motivate them to recover unless they are eligible for disability compensation. Studies consistently find that backache patients who receive compensation for their disability are significantly less likely to return to work than are patients who do not get any financial assistance.

This finding must be treated gingerly. It does NOT mean that people who claim to suffer backache are merely faking, or that the pain is all "in their head," or that unconsciously they want to stay hurt. Despite the widespread charge of malingering, we have no cause to doubt that people who say they want to recover *do* want to get better and that people who say they hurt really are in pain. But getting better calls for more than wanting.

Recovery calls for action on the part of the sufferer. In turn, action requires some emotional motivation. Usually pain itself will supply the motivation. Acute pain is precisely that—a call to action that will end the pain. Victims of chronic pain, however, have run out of things to do to ease their pain. No action seems to work; the pain persists. Eventually pain ceases to motivate. Any remaining urge to recover persists because people remember the old days and want to reclaim their lives. But where is the motivation if your life did not seem so great anyway and now your financial obligations are at least minimally taken care of?

Another group of patients lie at exactly the opposite end of the spectrum. They cannot wait to get back to their lives and jobs. Unfortunately, their jobs carry plenty of emotional stress. To recover and stay recovered they must find ways of relieving the stress that pervades their lives. Their challenge is not passivity; they are active, but they need to be creative enough to find a way to relax. Anxiety does not undermine them, but they need to find the courage to rethink their way of living. Depression does not vex them either, but they need the imagination to see an active life that is not dominated by tension. Creativity, courage, and imagination are common to us all, but they require confidence. And, as we saw in the example of the passenger in the car, unrelieved stress undermines confidence. So when the crisis comes and the back continues to hurt without respite, the overachiever faces as much danger of chronic pain as the underappreciated clerk. Ebenezer Scrooge and Bob Cratchit were both at risk for chronic back pain.

As a first step toward gaining confidence and a sense of control, most Americans try to learn what is wrong with their backs, but—as we shall see in the next chapter—this ambition is not so easily satisfied.

FINDING OUT WHAT'S WRONG

If you are like nine out of ten back sufferers, you will never learn *exactly* what is wrong with your back. Many complain, "I saw five specialists and each one gave me a different diagnosis." This uncertainty may seem disheartening, but usually it is the best sign because it can indicate that your backache does not arise from disease, nerve damage, or structural deformity. Doctors can usually agree on the nature of the problem when it is diseases, nerves, or damage, but if they can't, something else is wrong. You have suffered some form of soft-tissue damage. Perhaps you strained a muscle that was too tense or maybe you sprained a ligament. Damage of this sort does not show up on X rays and frankly it baffles most doctors.

Some patients become obsessed with obtaining a precise diagnosis. They become regular doctor shoppers, going from one to another in hopes of finding the one who knows the name of their particular problem. This attitude is not foolish, but for back trouble it is usually inappropriate. Modern medicine has become a marvel largely by virtue of proper diagnosis. Doctors can trace an ailment to a precise cause and then they treat exactly that problem. We are so used to the idea of medicine working this way that medical insurance in the United States demands a diagnosis before paying a claim. But backache seldom allows for such an on-the-button identification. Fortunately, knowing what to do for back problems seldom requires knowing exactly what is wrong. (Do not worry that the vagueness of the diagnosis will block your insurance. It can complicate a claim for disability compensation, but doctors know how to fill out an insurance form for ordinary back attacks. Often they list a suitably vague but scholarly name for unexplained back pain.)

This book's organization reflects the typical stages of a common back attack. No matter what the precise cause of the problem, your condition probably falls into one of these categories:

- *acute, or crisis, stage:* Pain is severe and sharp. Movement always carries the risk of pain; perhaps this pain is so great that you become frozen where you stand. You might find your body twisted into odd shapes by the attack. This stage usually is short-lived, lasting no more than two or three weeks. During this period you need to overcome the initial trauma and regain at least minimal strength for movement. Most people also want professional reassurance that their problem is a typical back attack.

- *recovery stage:* The worst is over but sudden pains can return at any moment and discomfort may be a regular part of life. This stage can last for several months, but should not continue for more than half a year. The worst of it should be over after three months. During this period you need to recover your strength, reflect on any aspects of your life that may have helped induce the attack, and put an end to the recurring pain. Professional help at this stage should provide temporary relief from your backache AND show you how to speed your own recovery.

- *latent, or well-back, stage:* Your back seems fine and you want to avoid the return of the problem. This stage may last the rest of your life, especially if you learn how to handle back stress. During this stage you can apply and develop the practices learned during the recovery period. Professionals for this stage are like coaches. They can help keep you on track, as needed.

- *chronic stage:* Something has gone wrong; the sufferer has become struck in the pain cycle and is not recovering. Most people want to move from chronic backache straight to the well-back stage, but real life does not work that way. The aim during chronic backache is to return to the recovery stage and resume the healing process. Professional help should focus on resolving the problems that have gotten the patient stuck.

Of course life is seldom as tidy as a book. The timetable given above will vary with each person. Recovery can slow down and lapses are also possible. Some unlucky patients undergo a second crisis during the recovery period.

THE COMMON BACKACHE

It takes several strategically placed mirrors to get a good look at your own back, so instead of peeking, imagine what your back looks like. Have you conjured up the picture of a skeleton's backbone or the shadows of an X ray? If so, you are making the same mistake that even some practictioners make. Reach behind you with your hand and feel your back. You can trace a line with your finger along your spine. Follow that line down toward your lower back. Coming off from either side of this line you can feel arches and curves, some hard, others soft. Use your sense of touch to understand your back. The bones of the spine are only a small part of the whole. Mostly your back is composed of the muscles and ligaments you have just examined.

Put your hand on your lower back again. Now move your back a little. If you are up to it, pump your back forward and backward. (Do nothing that hurts!) You can feel the different muscles acting in different ways. They work individually but in harmony.

With your right hand flat against the skin of your lower back, hold out your left hand in front of you and gently move it in a circle. You should be able to feel some mild motions in your back. These ripples show your back adjusting to the actions of your arm. Medicine still knows very little about the details of these interactions. Doctors only know that almost every activity produces harmonic adjustments in the back.

If anything goes wrong with this physical harmony, your back will reflect the problem. A muscle in this system may become strained, too tense or too weak to keep up its share of the performance. A spinal ligament may have stretched too far for proper responsiveness. Sometimes the problem is even more subtle. All your muscles may be fine, but some are overdeveloped. They are stronger, and the other, normal muscles cannot respond with equal strength. Athletes in splendid condition are subject to this type of strain. Over time the entire back will compensate for these local imbalances. You may feel the change as a twinge, as a persistent discomfort, or as a sudden piercing pain that results from some ordinary motion like standing up. Sometimes the results can be comical, or they would be if they were not so painful and frightening. It becomes impossible to sit or stand in a normal upright position. Muscle spasms can twist the body into a grotesque position.

Alarming as these imbalances are, they are NOT signs that your bones have slipped into some new and dreadful position. Perhaps only one muscle or ligament is in trouble, but your entire back is trying to compensate for this change. With so many muscles contorted, it is no easy matter to determine which one is hurt and which ones have simply adjusted to the shift in balance.

Why should an adaptive response hurt? Along with those muscles, ligaments, and bones, the back is rich in nerves. One of their normal functions is to trigger appropriate muscle actions to changing body positions. The nerves in your back, for example, signal the appropriate response to changes in hand position. Sometimes a nerve may be damaged directly, but more often the problem is subtle. Your nerves are fine, but they are signaling that your muscles are in a strange position. The details of these signals remain a mystery, but the result is clear enough. We experience pain.

Most people with backache suffer from some form of soft-tissue change that has brought on many adjustments by normal tissues. The nervous system detects these adjustments and we perceive them as pain.

Medicine still knows only the barest outline of how the muscles of the back perform their ballet, so a doctor is not going to have an easy time determining just what is wrong. Muscle movements and nervous signals do not show up in the X rays. The muscle spasms are likely to be obvious to the doctor, but their visibility does not lead to a ready explanation of why they are acting as they do.

In short, your whole system is in crisis. Distinguishing cause from effect clearly enough to say which problem triggered the others is no longer possible. Even if it could be done, the finding would be only of historical interest because treating the original problem won't alleviate the pain. Now you need to treat the whole system.

THE USES OF THE BACK

The back is not an organ like the lungs or liver, but is a system composed of bones, muscles, ligaments, and nerves. The bones of the back, known as vertebrae, run from the base of the skull to the coccyx, or tailbone. The neck consists of the first seven vertebrae of the spine. These bones pivot more than ordinary vertebrae to allow extensive turning of the head. Sometimes they can be forced far beyond their normal range, resulting in strangely persistent pain. Below the neck bone are the twelve vertebrae of the thoracic, or mid-body, spine. The ribs are attached to these vertebrae and this system is nearly immobile. That stability encourages the extra mobility of the neck. Lower still are the five large vertebrae of the lumbar spine, or lower-back region. Most back pain is in this area. The lumbar area is subject to sudden motion and to weight stresses that routinely bring enormous compressive and shearing forces against the spine and muscles. Together these regions of the back serve four major functions, which immediately become apparent to anyone who suffers a back attack.

LOAD BEARING. The spine is an architectural feature of the body with the same role that steel I beams play in skyscrapers or the buttress wall plays in a dam. If the I beams buckle or the buttress cracks, the structure collapses. The human body, too, is subject to compressive forces pushing down on the spine. These forces concentrate on the lumbar vertebrae of the lower back. In response the bones of the lower back are thicker and stronger, just like the lower part of the buttress for a dam. A person suffering through the acute stage of a back attack loses this load-bearing function and must lie down as much as possible. In a common back attack, load bearing is the first function to return.

MOBILITY. Unlike skyscrapers and dams, people must move about. That need explains why the "backbone" is really a series of distinct vertebrae rather than one long bone. We need all those joints to move easily. If the back's architecture were as rigid as a skyscraper's, we would be permanently upright. Our backs must permit all the stretching, bending over, and twisting that accompanies walking, crawling, and swimming. The back's supple functioning fails during a back attack and returns only after the recovery of its load-bearing ability.

CONTROL. What movement a person can muster during a back crisis is usually clumsy and mechanical. Sometime when your back is in good shape, try moving your arms while keeping your back perfectly rigid. You will discover that the easiest way to stay still is to imagine you are a robot and that your arm swings mechanically from a hinge at the shoulder joint. Human motion calls for help from the back. It is even more difficult to use your legs when your back is rigid. If you want to face in a new direction, you must turn with your feet like a soldier on parade. Control disappears during backache's crisis stage; expect nothing better than stiff motion. This function takes the longest to recover. Occasional stiff motion is to be expected even several months after the attack began.

HOUSING. Through the middle of the vertebrae runs the spinal cord, the link between your brain and the rest of the body. It is as crucial a passageway as the jugular vein and the windpipe. Damage to the spinal cord usually requires a major trauma, such as a bullet wound or terrible fall. More often at risk is the functioning of a nerve that emerges from the spinal cord to control some muscles. Many such nerves emerge from the lower back. Sometimes a strained muscle or ruptured disk will press against a nerve, causing intense pain. During a back crisis, however, you should not suffer a loss of nerve function. If your arms or legs become weak or immobile, see a doctor immediately. If your back attack began because of a sharp blow, you are not suffering a common backache. You should see your doctor at once.

FREQUENTLY CITED TROUBLES

A back attack arises from a loss of some or all back function. As we saw, strains, sprains, and muscular imbalances account for most back problems, but they are not the only causes. They are not even the best-known causes. Some of the most common explanations for back-ache are listed below.

"SLIPPED," RUPTURED, OR HERNIATED DISKS. One famous source of back pain is the so-called slipped disk. Disks are a natural form of padding placed between each vertebra, or spinal bone, and are critical to maintaining the back's mobility function. Disks are flexible, jellylike organs that bend and move with the motion of the spine. Their use is similar to the O rings made famous by the explosion of the *Challenger* space shuttle. In that accident we saw how tragic consequences may follow if an O ring does not respond properly to the physical stress of lift-off. Spinal disks can be overwhelmed by physical stress. Some-times a disk will weaken and sometimes it will even rupture. If the disk weakens, a back sufferer will lose some mobility and control. If the disk ruptures, the back's critical housing function may be at risk. If a disk bursts and spills its contents, fragments may press against a nerve. In this condition you may need surgery or some other medical procedure. Yet, for all its fame, the dam-aged disk constitutes an extreme minority of causes for lower-back pain. No more than 10 percent of back prob-lems arise from disk problems and most damaged disks do not rupture. Such is the renown of this diagnosis, however, that most people seem to assume that when their back suddenly aches they must have "slipped a disk."

SPINAL MISALIGNMENT. Chiropractors often say that a backache results from a misalignment of the vertebrae. Doctors, for their part, almost never agree that this is the problem, and they add that if your spine were to slip out of line, a chiropractor's manipulations would not be enough to correct the problem. Surgeons report that even when a patient is on the operating table and the spine lies open to direct manipulation, it is difficult for a doctor to move the spine. To support their diagnosis, chiropractors will point to an X ray and say that it shows the misalignment. Doctors viewing the same X ray usually say the spine is normal. An observer with ties to neither camp might note, however, that the manipulations of chiropractors have been used for several thousand years. X rays are a modern way of justifying an ancient technique. The diagnosis may be incorrect, but that does not mean the manipulations are worthless. Spinal manipulation, especially in its more gentle forms, helps many people who have not suffered damage to the nervous system.

WHIPLASH. Lawyers, more than doctors, favor this diagnosis. It is a general term for pain associated with the neck part of the spine and commonly arises when the neck stretches too far. Perched as it is above the stable vertebrae of the ribs, the neck may bend too far in response to a sudden body blow. Whiplash can result in a severe loss of neck mobility and control. If the neck pain extends down an arm, a neck disk may be involved in the injury. The pain of whiplash and lower backache both hurt far longer than medical theory can explain.

SCIATICA. There are many names for unexplained back discomfort, and sciatica is among the oldest. The word even turns up in Shakespeare. *Lumbago* is another word for that pain, as is *rheumatism*, although use of the latter is not limited to back cases. Historically, lumbago was back pain that stayed in the lower back. Sciatica was pain that continued from the back into the hips and legs. Pain continuing down the legs often reflects damage to a nerve, whereas the lumbago-type backache implies no risk to the back's housing of the central nervous system. The term "sciatica" is still in use among backache sufferers, although most doctors consider it an old-fashioned way of diagnosing a damaged disk. Doctors today have many terms available for back pain. A traditionalist may like sciatica for its age and Latin origins. Others can turn to more recent coinages, like *fibrositis*, although it, too, is now considered a bit old-fashioned. Many contemporary diagnoses begin with the word *idiopathic*, meaning unexplained. Other doctors favor a blunt English phrase like "lower back syndrome." None of these diagnoses identifies a specific ailment, however, and each may be considered translations of what the patient originally told the doctor, "My back hurts and I don't know why."

ARTHRITIS. There are many kinds of arthritis, a general term for soreness in the joints. Arthritis in the spine does account for some serious back disorders, although it is less common than a ruptured disk. Like a "slipped disk," spinal arthritis is feared and suspected more than it is experienced. Doctors see many people who arrive saying they have terrible arthritis in their back, but close examination shows this is not the case. Arthritis itself can take so many forms and is such a special case that it cannot be discussed at length here. Do not, however, accept a neighbor's suggestion that you probably have arthritis. Most back problems are not due to any form of spinal arthritis.

SPONDYLITIS. Occasionally a patient will receive a specific and unexpected diagnosis. Spondylitis, for example, is an inflammation of the spine. It cannot be treated in the same way an ordinary painful back sprain would be treated. Instead of listing these many rare conditions here, they have been included in the "Ready Reference" at the end of this book. Needless to say, anyone who has a specific disease of the back is not suffering the typical back attack discussed here. Because a backache may signal the onset of a serious and medically recognizable condition, it is often a good idea to see a doctor when your back starts to ache so that these conditions can be ruled out. Paradoxically, these rare conditions are often easier for a doctor to treat than the common (and less dangerous) backache.

LIVING WITH
A VAGUE DIAGNOSIS

Instead of looking for the specific cause of their hurt, most patients are wiser to work on regaining as much of their life as possible. Usually a patient can recover all that was important, including such back-stressing sports as playing tennis and horseback riding. Lasting recovery, however, almost always means making some changes in your way of living. Chase out the unrelieved stress; get your diet straight; get your muscles into better shape; make pleasure a regular part of your day, and enjoy the sense of being recalled to life.

No doctor, chiropractor, or faith healer can make those changes for you. So even if you are lucky enough to find a true wonder worker, you are still the one in charge and still the one responsible for the outcome of your case. Of course this does not mean you should exclude therapists from your recovery. They are important, but they are helpers. Consider the example of this story told by a former backache victim:

I used to have chronic neck, shoulder, and upper back pain, with some pain now and then in my lower back. Nothing really alleviated it, including chiropractic (although that did help some). [Then a friend recommended a man] who teaches some kind of combination yoga exercises and heaven-knows-what-else plus he would do chiropractic adjustments along the entire spine and neck after the two-hour exercise class. Inside of two weeks, I could not only turn my head with ease but was pain-free for the first time in about ten years—and the effects have lasted. I still do the exercises from time to time when I feel myself tightening up again. These exercises also eliminated the lower back pain I'd been experiencing—which he contended was responsible for all the tension in my upper back and neck.

. . . [The experience] showed me that I could do something about this by myself—that I didn't need to be passive and have someone else, say a chiropractor, do something for me.

This story has a happy ending, but it is a shame that this woman took years to learn it was her responsibility to put an end to back pain. Today she shows a healthy attitude. If the pain returns, she knows what she can do about it herself.

The special problems of backache call for special responses. Instead of focusing your energy on finding out what is wrong, you should concentrate on moving as quickly as possible through the stages of back misery to full recovery. As you seek professional advice remember that, more than a specific diagnosis, you need to find out what to do. This idea is as strange to many practitioners as it is to patients.

Traditional health professionals see themselves as healers, not teachers. This view helps explain the shocking statistic found by one survey that only 13 percent of doctors and 26 percent of other practitioners recommended an exercise procedure to their back patients. Exercises are the key to quick recovery. But since exercises are the patient's responsibility, healers may not see teaching the exercises as part of their job. Most backache professionals can relieve your pain temporarily, but temporary relief becomes chronic pain if you do not progress toward recovery. Backache is not one of those conditions that benefits from the advice to continue with the medication for another week and see what happens. You have to make something happen.

THREE

OVERCOMING THE CRISIS: BACKACHE IN THE ACUTE STAGE

There is a maneuver every backache sufferer should know and be ready to use whenever a back attack threatens:

Emergency knee hug:

Lie on your back with your knees bent. Pull your knees as close to your chest as you can. Hug them tightly with your arms and hold that position for five minutes. If this position is too painful, lie on your side and tuck your knees up toward your chest. Hold them for five minutes.

This action stretches and relaxes the muscles of your back. It is a first-aid measure that can avert or lessen many a crisis. Use it when you feel your back is *beginning* to give you trouble.

Many people dismiss the first stirrings of back pain. They press on until the attack becomes so acute, they can barely move. The first rule of backache is: Take your back seriously. You may tell yourself that the pain you just endured was "nothing," or was just a momentary twinge, or that you can take it. Lying on the floor for five minutes in an emergency knee hug may seem like an overreaction to a moment's sharp sting, but that sting warned of trouble. Normal movements should not bring pain, not even flashes of them.

STEP ONE:
REST YOUR BACK

If you have suddenly developed a piercing pain that cannot be abolished by an emergency knee hug, you are suffering an acute attack. Acute attacks can also begin with a few warning aches that quickly—within a few days—develop into agony. The first step toward ending this crisis is to get off your back. Lie down on a bed. If you cannot—or dare not—move, lie on the floor and get to your bed as soon as you can. Put a pillow under your knees to lift and slightly flex the muscles. This position takes pressure off the sciatic nerve. If you cannot tolerate this position or feel you must move, lie on your side with your knees drawn partially up toward your chest.

Physicians tend to say you should get to a hospital immediately. Kinesiologists also recommend an emergency visit to their office. Generally, however, this trip can be delayed. If you have no history of kidney trouble and your back pain came in response to some ordinary action, resting your back usually is more important than seeing a doctor at once. Take the load off your back and stay still. Plan on spending the rest of this day in bed. If you can get a bedpan, so much the better. It is best to limit any movement.

In these days of supermedications, it seems only natural to take a powerful painkiller. The best medication for backache, however, is one of the most common. Aspirin generally does the trick. It has fewer side effects than prescription drugs and is an effective source of temporary relief. If surgery is under consideration for your case, stronger pain medication is advisable. Any doctor will almost automatically prescribe something stronger than aspirin for an acute back attack, but do not suppose you must run to a doctor in order to get a prescription. Over-the-counter pain relief can usually ease the discomfort enough to lie still in bed. If aspirin and lying still does not reduce the pain, get a prescription for a stronger painkiller. In this case a narcotic prescription is justified, for the importance of reducing the pain outweighs the slight risk of addiction.

The bad news about pain is that it is going to be with you for a time. The worst of it should subside within a few weeks, or perhaps even in a few days, but you are still likely to feel occasional sharp aching several months from now. Do not suppose that you are resting to let the pain go away. You are lying down just to recover your back's functions of load bearing, mobility, and control. The pain that sent you to bed indicates that your back's capacity to function has given way. The pain will not disappear until after you have restored your functioning. That unfortunate principle means you are going to get to know your pain quite intimately.

Besides lying down and taking aspirin, it is a good idea to put a compress on the aching area. Some people favor cold compresses; others advocate heat. If your backache came as an immediate response to some motion or other, chances are good that you have strained a muscle. In this case moist heat can serve as a relaxant. An easy way to apply moist heat is with a wet towel. A gadget known as a hydrocollator can also serve. It is a canvas bag filled with sand. Soak it in hot water and wrap a towel around it. The dry heat from an electric heating pad can sometimes cause strained muscles to lock in a spasm.

If your backache came on suddenly, perhaps shortly after some vigorous activity, you may have torn a ligament or muscle. The tear itself probably was too small to hurt immediately, but internal bleeding has led to a backache. In that case heat only aggravates the condition because it increases the circulation. Use a cold compress instead to stop the swelling. An ice pack on the lower back may soothe the discomfort. Another procedure is to put ice on the back for an hour. Then use moist heat for an hour, and then return to the ice.

If you are not sure whether to try ice or heat first, try ice. And don't stop with the ice after the first two days. Use it regularly during the acute stage.

When pain is constant seeking some pleasure is a necessity. Although you are not yet ready for even a gentle massage, soft stroking and rubbing of your back can help. Have someone you care about rub a balm or ointment on your back. That shared intimacy is preferable to rubbing it on yourself. The physical relief offered by such medication is, at best, only mild and temporary, but you need reminders that relief is possible and pain has not taken over the world. Don't try to tough it out; indulge yourself a little.

Introduce the visualization technique (discussed in the opening chapter) on your first day in bed and keep it up throughout both the acute stage and the recovery period. The other stress-reduction techniques described in the first chapter—drinking water, shrugging shoulders, and maintaining a diary—should not begin until the third day.

The second day should usually be spent in bed as well. Begin the day with an emergency knee hug. Then lie flat again, with that pillow under your knees. Late in the afternoon of your second day you can begin to assess the seriousness of your problem. Do you have a temperature? Has your back attack been accompanied by bladder or bowel difficulties? If the answer to either question is yes, your backache may result from a duodenal ulcer or from some kidney trouble. It is smart practice to see a doctor, just to make sure that your backache is not a symptom of some more dangerous problem. If you have other symptoms as well as back pain, you definitely should arrange to see a doctor.

The second part of your self-evaluation is to do a stretch test. Discover which motions you can make without pain.

STRETCH TESTS

The first time you give yourself a stretch test, do it while lying in bed. Later, if it seems possible, do the tests while lying on the floor. You can have a pillow under your head if you like. Keep another pillow under your knees. Let pain be your guide. Push yourself if you simply feel tired or weak, but do not continue with an exercise that hurts too much.

Test 1: This is a simple breathing exercise.

a. Expel all the air from your lungs. Push your stomach down with your hands to help the air out.

b. Hold your breath; count slowly to three.

c. Inhale slowly through your nose.

d. Hold your breath; count slowly to three.

e. Exhale.

This test gives you an exaggerated feel for the breathing that you will use during the other stretch tests. Breathing is an important part of every exercise. Normally you should not hold your breath during an exercise, but it is advised as part of these stretch tests.

Test 2:

a. Rest your arms out straight from your sides.

b. As you inhale slowly through your nose, lift your arms, keeping them straight, until they are slightly higher than your head.

c. Count slowly to three.

d. Exhale fully and drop arms to your side.

e. On a scale of one to ten, rate the pain involved in that stretch.

If you rated the pain as less than five, repeat the exercise. This time raise your arms a bit higher. Keep going through this cycle until you either find it too painful or you have your arms so far above the head that the hands touch.

FURTHER TESTS: Repeat the procedure of stretch Test 2 using the following motions in Step B (the inhale step):

- Bend your knees and pull them up until your heels touch the pillow beneath your knees.

- Push your head up and raise your upper body until you lean back on a 45-degree angle. (Note: Push up with your outstretched arms. Do not pull up with your back muscles.)

- Roll over on your right side.

- Roll over on your left side.

- Shrug your shoulders.

These stretch tests and the pain ratings you score each one will give you a good sense of how you stand and how you are progressing. Do not be alarmed if, at the beginning, these simple moves prove to be too painful to endure. Backache has a shocking ability to block even the simplest actions you once took for granted. Do these tests at least twice a day. You should see steady progress in your capacity to do them. The progress is a more important guide to your condition than the amount of pain at the outset. Shrugging shoulders is a stress-reduction technique (see the first chapter). Once you know you can do it without pain, develop it as a way to reduce stress.

STEP TWO:
RESTORE THE LOAD FUNCTION

Traditionally, doctors favored a long bed-rest period after a back attack. More recent wisdom says to get going after only one or two days in bed. On the *third day* you will find that your motion is still severely restricted, but now is the time to start recovering the functions you have lost. The most basic function is supporting the body's weight. Even if mobility is still difficult, you should get out of bed and stand up. Treat the action like a stretch test. Exhale. Inhale through the nose while forcing yourself into a sitting position. Rest and exhale. Inhale through the nose and stand up. Exhale. If you can stand still without much pain, your back is showing signs of improvement. The load-bearing function is returning.

If you can move about, get rid of the bedpan. The trek to the bathroom will be good for you. Start drinking eight glasses of water per day as an antistress technique (see Chapter 1). Do your stretch tests while lying on the floor.

Another important technique is to maintain a diary or log of your activities. On a sheet of paper write down what you are doing every half hour. Keep it up throughout the day. If you move about, carry the paper with you. At the end of the day it should look something like the example opposite. You can see that the day was not terribly busy. More important, the backache sufferer can see the same thing. One important use of the log is to motivate its keeper. Diaries show backache sufferers just how limited their lives have become. A second use is as a source of reassurance. They provide visible evidence of how much a person has improved. On the sample log, for example, you can see that by the end of the day standing was becoming a common activity. The back's load-bearing function is returning. During the acute stage of your back problem you should maintain a log of each day, starting with the third day.

During this crisis stage you should not sit down. Sitting is much harder on the back than is standing. The common expression "Sit down, take a load off your feet" tells only half the truth. Sitting does reduce the load on your feet; however, it transfers that load straight to the back. Avoid sitting as much as possible. Lie down or stand up during this acute phase. If you have paperwork to do, spread it on the floor and lie down. If you want to eat with others who are at a table, stand up to eat. Lie on your side to read. Lie down or stand up to watch television. If you must sit up, do it in bed while fully propped up with pillows, and lean back into the pillows. Let them support your weight.

LOG OF DAY'S ACTIVITIES
Date: Saturday Oct. 14, 1989

9:00   *Stretch tests—hardest was sitting up*

9:30   *Resting*

10:00   *Shower*

10:30   *Resting*

11:00

11:30

12:00

12:30   *Light lunch—slept through last several log periods*

1:00   *Drink water*

1:30   *Walking around*

2:00   *Lie on floor listening to television*

2:30   *Still listening to television*

3:00   *In bed—drinking water*

3:30

4:00

4:30   *Slept through last log periods—awakened by call from Bob*

5:00   *Stretch test—sat up better*

5:30   *Standing up watching news on TV*

6:00   *Lying on floor listening to TV*

6:30   *Standing to eat light supper*

STEP 3:
RESTORE MOBILITY

Exercise is an essential part of reducing back pain and getting moving again. Once you can stand up without pain, even if standing straight is still difficult, you should begin exercises to restore elasticity to your muscles. Begin with the stretch tests as warm-ups and relaxers. In these first days be careful not to overdo the exercises. If an exercise increases your pain, stop it. Do not hold your breath. Proper breathing is important, but since it is difficult to learn an exercise and to breathe properly at the same time, we shall first discuss the exercise, then the breathing.

Pelvic Exercise:

a. Lie on floor (a carpeted floor is perfectly okay) with a pillow under your knees. Bend the knees enough to get feet flat on the floor. You may have a thin pillow under your head if you wish.

b. Slip your right hand under the arch in your back so that your fingers can feel the spine.

c. Place your left hand on your stomach and feel the stomach with your palm.

d. Slowly tighten your buttocks as hard as you can.

e. When the muscles are tightened hold them and count to five.

f. Relax the muscles.

Once you have learned the basic actions of the exercise, it is time to get the breathing right:

1. Inhale through nose as you tighten buttocks.

2. Exhale slowly through mouth as you count to five, keeping your buttocks tight.

3. Exhale as you relax your buttocks.

The major muscles used in this exercise are the gluteals, the muscles that are most important in limiting the sway of your back as you walk or run. As you did the exercise you should have felt your back pushing down on your right hand, and your left hand should have felt the stomach muscles tighten.

g. Repeat steps *a* through *f*, breathing correctly.

h. When you can comfortably do steps *a–f* 10 times, change step *e*. As you count to five and exhale raise your head above the floor. At this stage of your back attack you should not lift the shoulders.

Relaxation Exercise:

a. Resume basic position: lie flat on floor, pillow under knees, knees bent enough to permit feet to be flat on floor.

b. Place both hands on stomach, palms down.

c. Relax stomach so you can feel a basin between your ribs and pubic area.

d. Pull your head back so there is plenty of space between shoulders and ears; look toward knees, not at ceiling.

e. Inhale slowly through the nose while keeping stomach in.

f. Exhale slowly through the mouth while keeping stomach in.

g. Let hands fall to side and relax.

This exercise is a basic one for the early days of recovering mobility.

Leg Lifts:

a. Resume basic position flat on floor, but without pillow under knees.

b. Roll onto right side, with back of left hand feeling your back.

c. Tense your body.

d. Slowly raise left leg.

e. Slowly lower left leg.

f. Relax body and roll onto back.

When you know the basic maneuvers use this breathing system:

1. Inhale as you roll onto side.

2. Exhale as you raise your leg.

3. Inhale as you lower your leg.

4. Exhale when you roll onto your back.

After you have mastered the breathing you can add a further step:

g. Roll onto left side and repeat maneuver.

After the leg lifts do another relaxation exercise.

These gentle exercises may prove shockingly difficult to perform. Do not push yourself beyond your pain. Imagine your pain as a stern teacher, letting you know quickly what is and what is not within your limits, and listen to your teacher. By touching your back and stomach as you do the exercises you gain immediate knowledge of what happens when you move. The simple motions you have always taken for granted are not so simple after all.

Do these exercises and the stretch tests twice a day. As you grow stronger steadily reduce the amount of time you spend lying in bed. Do not yet begin to sit down, but increase your time spent standing. Your pain will persist, but it should ease. Remember that the goal at this stage of your back attack is to recover basic back functioning. Ending the pain takes longer.

If you were exercising regularly before the back crisis, you can usually resume simple swimming after five days. (This timetable assumes that your exercises have progressed well.) Be sure not to arch your back as you swim. If on the fifth day the idea of getting out of bed still seems too painful to contemplate, see a doctor. Rest, ice, and medication should have helped by now. Do not develop a patient attitude toward pain.

Sometimes a back's load-bearing capacity fails because of sprained ligaments. Each vertebra is kept in place by a series of ligaments that have the primary role in supporting stretching loads. If stretched too far or for too long, one or more ligaments may sprain. Particularly at risk are the iliolumbar ligaments, triangular-shaped ligaments attached to the lowest lumbar vertebra and the pelvis. They are important in keeping the base of the spine pointed straight up and are a common site of strain. An exercise for people who are having difficulty standing erect is the *lateral trunk stretch*. Insert this exercise into your twice-daily regimen of exercises:

a. Begin with basic position: lying flat on back and feet flat, but with NO PILLOW under your knees.

b. Put your hands behind your head.

c. Cross your right leg over your left leg, just above the left knee.

d. Press your left knee to the floor, using the right leg to hold it in place.

e. Shift your lower left leg as far to the right as you can without feeling pain. (Use the weight of your right leg to hold the upper part of the left leg in place.)

f. Count to five. You can feel the stretch along the right side of your spine.

g. Uncross your legs and relax.

The breathing to accompany this exercise works this way:

1. Exhale as you press your leg to the right and count to five.

2. Inhale as you uncross your legs to return to the starting position.

h. Repeat the exercise, this time pinning your right leg with your left.

Try to do this exercise five times, to start with. At first you may find that you cannot do the exercise at all elegantly. For example, you may not be able to press one or both knees to the floor without straining too much. Do what you can as sloppily as you must. Your goal is to get so that you can do ten proper stretches. This exercise stretches tightened muscles on either side of the spine. They must work in harmony for you to stand up straight.

SURVIVING THE CRISIS

For about three quarters of backache sufferers the crisis period ends within ten days to three weeks. The pain eases but does not disappear entirely, and there is no absolute moment when we can say the crisis has passed.

For the purposes of this book we will say the crisis ends when your back regains its basic load-bearing and movement functions. The program described in this chapter should help you recover the ability to stand up straight and to move about, even if your movement is still awkward.

If just standing up remains painful, the problem may be more than soft-tissue damage. Load bearing is managed by several parts of the back. The vertebrae support the weight, and the disks support the vertebrae. Sometimes the compressive forces pushing down on the disk cause it to bulge and press on a nerve. An especially serious symptom of nerve pressure is pain that runs down the leg from the back and continues on below the knee. If pain persists BELOW the knee, you should bring that fact to the attention of an orthopedist or neurologist.

During the acute stage it is important to overcome any long-term fears for your back. The principle is the same as the old adage that tells a person who falls off a horse to climb back in the saddle immediately. If your back crisis began with some simple motion like standing up to reach for a test booklet, or carrying a tray to a table, or bending over to tie a shoe, or any other normal action, you should try to repeat the action as soon as you can. Thus, if your attack began when you bent to tie your shoe, bend over and tie your shoe. You should not try it on the first day, or even the third day, but do it once you recover your ability to stand up straight and move about. Be careful. Make it a little easier for yourself. Set your foot on something so you do not have to bend to the floor. (You should always do that anyway, even when your back is fine.) Now tie your shoe. The particular action that triggered a back attack was not really the cause. The real problem lay in the tension and stresses of your back. The trigger was just a chance stress, and anything could have set your back off. Easy to say. But emotionally it is not so easy to believe. Once you see that you can do the action, however, your fears can begin to subside.

If the body were logical, the end of the crisis would

mean the end of the pain. You have recovered your back's main functions, and instead of easing off the back, you should exercise it plenty. But there is no logic in the body. It will continue to hurt, intermittently, for some time. If you want to see a doctor, do not feel you should wait until the pain resumes. Anyone who works with backs knows that off-and-on pain is more the rule than the exception. Backache generally reflects old habits that restrict the back's flexibility. That limitation may reflect persistent tension that comes from unresolved emotional stress, or it may simply reflect years of inactivity. Muscles that go unused for long times can forget how to stretch normally. Once you overcome the crisis, you must still resolve the habits that brought you low in the first place.

HELP DURING
AN ACUTE ATTACK

If you see a doctor during the acute stage, you will probably be told to spend a few days in bed, put an ice pack on your painful spot, and take some pain medication. If you are told anything else, find out why. (Surgery is discussed in Chapter 7.) Ask twice if you are told to get into traction. The classic idea behind traction in a back attack is to pull the vertebrae apart and ease the compressive forces, but doctors now know that it takes too much force to separate the vertebrae and the patient cannot stand these forces. A second reason is for disciplinary purposes. A person who simply will not go to bed can be put in traction just to keep him still. If a doctor proposes traction, ask if bed rest will do just as well. Then go to bed and stay there for the next three days.

Many patients complain that the doctor they see first does not take an acute attack seriously, but you do not want your doctor to say, "The tests show you have such and such a disease." A baffled look and shrug of puzzlement are good signs in this case. It is good news when a doctor says the tests are inconclusive. Usually a practitioner will add some reassurances, but some doctors with a particularly unsatisfactory manner will say, "Nothing is wrong with you." Your back tells you that something *is* wrong, but the doctor's brusque dismissal of your pain means your problem is routine. Here are the types of doctors you can see for your back pain:

GENERAL PRACTITIONER (M.D.). The best place to begin is with your family doctor, if you have one. A GP who is willing to work with you is commonly the best doctor for this stage of your suffering. A GP can determine if there is a problem that needs to be chased down. But remember, you want a full examination. The point is to find out whether anything unusual is wrong, and that can be discovered only if you are examined in detail. A family doctor who responds to reports of a backache with an immediate recommendation for rest and a prescription for a painkiller is not doing you a favor. Ask for the name of a specialist. Be sure to add that you want a conservative doctor, one who is not too quick to advise surgery.

EMERGENCY-WARD DOCTOR (M.D.). People who do not have a family doctor may feel tempted to seek out an emergency room. This effort is seldom satisfactory, unless you suspect you have broken your back.[1] Emergency rooms will not carry out the full examination you need, and X rays almost never reveal anything abnormal.

ORTHOPEDISTS (M.D.). These doctors are the ones most likely to diagnose a ruptured disk. Specialists in the

---

[1] A broken back need not be as serious and terrifying as it sounds. Most people associate broken backs with fatal injuries or ones resulting in permanent paralysis. Many times, however, a fracture of the spine does not damage the spinal cord. If you hurt your back in a fall, do not rule out a fracture simply because you can move your legs and toes. Some people fracture their spines and never notice anything more than a bit of discomfort.

skeletal system may seem like the natural experts to turn to when your back hurts, but remember that most backache results from sprains and strains of soft tissue. A bone expert may not be able to do much in these cases. Some orthopedists will do spinal manipulations, but they seldom linger over patients whose X rays show nothing clear. Most orthopedists can help backache only in cases requiring surgery. Many patients complain about the way orthopedists cannot offer a precise diagnosis. Patients who recognize the difficulty in diagnosing ordinary back trouble, however, appreciate what the orthopedist has done: Confirm that the problem is an ordinary back attack, not a rare disease of the spine. The orthopedist has done exactly what the patient wants.

PHYSIATRIST (M.D.). The most satisfactory approach to the recovery stage of backache comes from the branch of medicine that specializes in physical rehabilitation. There are only about 3,000 physiatrists in the United States, and those who do exist are concentrated in the largest cities. Their numbers are growing rapidly, however. They have doubled since the early 1980s and are one of the most sought after residencies in America. Their success in backache arises from their wide-angle view of the patient. They treat people as a whole, combining body with mind. Their approach to physical recovery focuses on natural means, like heat and exercise, instead of drugs and surgery. (They do use medication to treat acute pain.) Physiatrists are not dismayed by the idea of soft-tissue injury and can explore the back by touch to determine the nature of many injuries other doctors cannot find. They also believe in psychology's contribution to physical health and recognize the role of emotional stress in backache.

KINESIOLOGIST. A chiropractor who has degrees in both chiropractics and kinesiology (the study of body movement) is superior to a plain and simple chiropractor.

Chiropractors specialize in manipulating the body. Their diagnosis for a backache typically is "subluxation," or spinal misalignment. Chiropractors get the lion's share of the backache-patient market, treating millions more patients for back pain than do medical doctors. Their popularity and ability to produce short-term relief through spinal manipulation irritates many medical doctors, but this success is not a fluke. The theory of chiropractics is relatively recent, but many of its manipulative and physical techniques for reducing pain were used by the ancient Greeks and Romans. The techniques are proven sources of short-term relief. A chiropractor who has also studied the anatomy and mechanics of body movement is better equipped to deal with your chronic back pain. You should look for a kinesiologist who is willing to talk to you about things you can do to help yourself. As a rule, kinesiologists and chiropractors are much more willing to discuss your pain and its relation to your whole life than are most medical specialists, but insurance can be a tricky issue with chiropractors. Most medical plans will pay for them, but some of the most popular ones do not. Government-financed medical insurance commonly allows such a small outlay per visit to a chiropractor that the practitioner has no time for more than the basic manipulations. You need to see a professional who has the time to show you exercises and to see that you do them correctly. A kinesiologist normally gives such care, but may not have the time to accept patients hoping to pay through government insurance.

FOUR

THE RECOVERY STAGE: RESTORING CONTROL

After the acute stage ends, backache sufferers still face two important problems. Their mobility remains limited, and they are still in pain. For many people the pain is the more serious problem, and much backache therapy given during this second stage focuses on ending pain. Technology and medication, in particular, aim at providing relief. Even some surgery tries simply to end the pain. Backache victims tell themselves that once the pain goes away, they will recover full mobility. Natural as this thinking seems, it has the clinical facts of backache exactly in reverse. By regaining full control over your movements, the pain will subside.

Backache sufferers as a group tend to be out of shape, stiff (especially in the trunk), and suffer from local muscle spasms. The pain reflects these conditions, and any treatment that ignores these parts of the problem is likely to prove temporary and partial. Persistent pain can be especially dismaying for people who think of their bodies as machines. They reason that if their equipment cannot function completely, it must still be broken; however, the human body is not really a mechanical device but a marvelously adaptive organism. The spine develops many bone spurs and outcroppings that appear in X ray after X ray, especially as people grow older. The conventional wisdom used to hold that these spurs were a nuisance and must be "pinching a nerve." Then people began to ask, "Why blame the spurs since they are an ordinary part of healthy backs as well as pained ones?" Contemporary research suggests that these growths are normal spinal adaptations to keep the back stable in the face of continuous stresses.

It helps to think of persistent backache as an unfortunate prolongation of an adaptation. Like the spine, the mind and its perceptions of the back also adapt. A person with acute backache becomes more alert to tensions and pains, thereby avoiding dangerous actions. When the back attack began this adaptation was valuable. You hurt yourself and should keep still. Now you seem better, yet it is as though your body remembers the pain and continues to fear it. You need to readapt your perceptions to your recovered healthy state. There is no free path to this readaptation, just as there is no free way to develop callouses. If you want to be a carpenter, you must go through a period when your hands are too soft for the job. If you want to reclaim your life, you must go through a period when your back is too tender.

The previous chapter advised you to let pain be your guide to the pace of your recovery. That advice was good for sufferers in an acute phase of back attack. During the recovery phase, however long it lasts, the advice must change a bit. Continue to let pain set the limits of your exercises, but do not let it define the limits to your ambitions. Pain cannot be your guide to getting off the sofa and on with your life. A recovery from backache usually mixes four approaches:

- *adaptation* of body positions to find new ways of doing old things;

- *relaxation* techniques to relieve muscle tension;

- *exercises* to stretch and strengthen muscles used in supporting the back;
- *temporary relief* from pain helps restore morale and gives a person occasion to do more than possible during periods of pain.

ADAPTING NORMAL ACTIVITY

Your diary of activities will show you how much of your life you have recovered and how far you have still to go. If you prefer, you can switch your diary keeping to a once-a-week activity, but really keep that log once a week. It is the best reminder you have for seeing how much the pain is taking out of your life. As you regain control your life should take on more of its normal character. In the meantime, adapt your style of behavior so you can recover as much activity as possible. Do not wait until you can do things in the old manner before you do them at all.

One important area that people are eager to reclaim is sex. Sexual intercourse calls for pelvic movements that may be extremely painful for a person with chronic lower backache. The so-called missionary position can be especially painful, particularly for the person on top. Look for other positions. Sufferers should not abandon sexual relations merely because they have a bad back, but fear can inhibit both partners. By adapting to the circumstances a good sex life can continue during chronic backache. If you find a proper position, sex may even benefit your back. The rhythmic motions, if kept gentle, are a mildly therapeutic exercise. Some people like lying on their sides, but this position can be painful too. In one position that can be more comfortable, the woman lies on her side, her knees pulled forward, and the man embraces her from behind, fitting his body to hers. The partner without backache can be the more vigorous in movement, but you may find that these movements are more like stretch exercises and can be done quite comfortably.

This search for the comfortable position is the basic idea behind restoring many other activities to your life during the chronic phase. Do you work behind a desk? Perhaps there is a better way to sit, or should you stand for a time? Does your work include difficult labor? You can look for better positions and for warm-up exercises that will get you into shape. (Do not try heavy lifting until your back has fully recovered.)

RELAXING DURING
PERSISTENT BACKACHE

During the acute phase relaxation meant getting plenty of bed rest. That stage has passed. A recovering backache sufferer should be up and about, but do not abandon a program of relaxation. Continue with your visualization exercises and with massages. Your massage partner still should stroke rather than knead the body. The object of the massage is simply pleasurable relaxation. Kneading may hurt a painful back.

Good backache therapists include relaxation techniques as part of their treatment. Relaxation training can teach techniques for keeping physical stress to a minimum while you work. It can also teach exercises for self-produced relaxation. The deep physical relaxation and increased self-awareness promoted by these exercises combine ideas from self-hypnosis, yoga, massage, and deep abdominal breathing. Chiropractors usually pay close attention to muscle relaxation. Physical therapists try to learn about you as well as about your back pain so that they can prescribe a suitable relaxation therapy. Physiatrists specialize in teaching natural methods of relaxing mind and body. Whichever method you use, begin with a therapist who can observe what you do and correct you.

Once you know how to do it, you can—if you like—exercise alone.

A couple of basic yoga breathing exercises can be mastered without the help of a guru. One simple relaxation exercise lets you stay in your chair.

a. Sit comfortably in a chair. Stretch your arms and legs, and lean against the backrest.

b. Close your eyes.

c. Purse your lips, making a narrow opening of the mouth to breathe through.

d. As you inhale roll your head back. Do not stretch the neck. The idea is simply to roll your head to a comfortable position.

e. As you exhale roll your head forward until your chin touches your body.

f. Repeat steps *d* and *e* at least five times.

Another classic relaxation exercise is a modification of the emergency knee hug. That emergency maneuver is for times when tension has grown enough to be threatening. On more normal occasions a simpler exercise will serve.

a. Lie on the floor, arms at your side.

b. Slowly raise and pull your right knee toward your chest.

c. Hug your knee.

d. Return your leg to floor.

e. Repeat steps *c* and *d* four more times.

f. Repeat steps *c* through *e*, using the left knee.

Breathing is critical to this exercise.

1. Exhale as you lie on floor.

2. Inhale as you draw your knee toward you.

3. Exhale as you hug your knee.

4. Inhale as you return your knee to floor.

Besides reducing stress, relaxation exercises go after the anxiety that worsens the effects of chronic backache. It is difficult to reclaim your life if you are continually afraid that an activity might hurt. Anxiety over pain is self-fulfilling. When we are anxious we tend to experience actions as painful that in more relaxed times would not hurt us.

EXERCISES TO RECOVER CONTROL

Exercise is a necessary part of almost every back recovery. Its purpose is to recover your body's flexibility, strength, endurance, and cardiovascular fitness. Back exercises are notoriously dull; they are more like warm-up exercises than like team games or gymnastics. The satisfaction these exercises can bring lies in the intimate acquaintance they give with your own body and its progress. As you work with the program you will become increasingly aware of your body. You will sense muscular tensions that you never noticed before. In time you will be able to say to yourself, "Hmm. My back seems to be tightening up," and you will know which exercises can help best. Growing body awareness is the foundation of a successful exercise program.

You can accompany your exercise program with music to help create a relaxed mood and to encourage graceful movement. The athletic saying "No pain, no gain" has no place in this exercise program. You should push yourself and have a sense of exertion, but exertion is not pain. Do not push an exercise to the point of hurting. If something does start to hurt, ease up on it. (Note: Sometimes exercise leads to aching after you stop. These aches come from stretching unused muscles and are not directly related to your backache.)

Do the following exercises twice a day:

Warm-ups

a. Lie on floor with a pillow under your head and your legs stretched out flat.

b. Inhale deeply through your nose.

c. Exhale slowly through your mouth.

d. Inhale deeply again and raise your arms slowly over your head.

e. Exhale again and slowly lower your arms to your sides.

f. Repeat steps *b* through *e* three more times.

g. Inhale deeply and tense entire body, making fists with both hands as you do.

h. Exhale slowly, releasing the body tension and fists as you do.

i. Repeat steps *g* and *h* three more times.

j. Inhaling through nose, pull your knees up to a bent position and get your feet flat on the floor.

k. Exhale through mouth.

l. Inhaling through nose, press your lower back down while raising your hips as far as you can.

m. Repeat steps *k* and *l* three more times.

n. Exhale, relaxing your back and slipping your feet forward to reach the original position.

Flexibility Exercises

Lower-back Stretch

a. Lie on back, head on pillow, knees bent, feet flat.

b. Pull right knee toward chest as far as you can.

c. Hold position to count of five.

d. Return foot to floor and wobble legs.

e. Repeat steps *b* through *d*, using the left knee.

Eventually you should be able to do this exercise ten times. Do no more than five at first. Once ten becomes easy, pull both legs at once. Breathe:

1. Inhale as you pull knee up.

2. Exhale during release.

Pelvic Stretch

a. Lying flat on back, pull knees up until feet are flat on floor. Keep knees together.

b. Keeping your back flat, swivel pelvis to right so that knees touch floor on left side.

c. Count to five.

d. Raise knees.

e. Repeat steps *b–d*, but swivel left and touch floor on right side.

Do this exercise three times to begin with. Keeping your back flat is more important than pressing knees all the way to the floor. Try to bring the number up to ten times. Breathe:

1. Inhale on step *a*.

2. Exhale during swivel.

3. Inhale during count.

Strengthening Exercises

Stomach Developer

Most people think of traditional high school sit-ups as the best stomach developers. Backache sufferers should use only a modified form of that exercise.

a. Do not lie on the floor. Sit on it. Keep your knees bent and feet flat on the floor. Pull your legs wide enough so that the inner sides of the knees are even with the hips.

b. Bend back toward the floor. Go only as far as you can without feeling pain, and do not go all the way back to a flat position. Keep your arms relaxed at your side. Let your stomach muscles do the work. Keep your feet flat on floor.

c. Before LOWER BACK touches floor hold your position and tense stomach muscles.

d. Count to five.

e. Pull yourself forward.

f. Repeat three more times.

At the start you may want to support yourself with your arms because you can barely bend back at all without falling backward. Don't use your arms any more than you can help. You will get better at it. You can use your inner thighs to help pull yourself back up and to help hold yourself as you count to five. With practice you will find that your thighs and stomach can do all the pulling.

The breathing pattern for this exercise:

1. Inhale as you check your position.

2. Exhale while you roll back.

3. Inhale when you pull forward.

Second Stomach Strengthener

The abdomen has the most important muscles for stabilizing the back. To develop the stomach muscles further, include a second partial sit-up in your program:

a. Lie down on floor without using a pillow. Let arms lie loosely by your side.

b. Pull your legs back so that the heels touch your thighs. Keep knees touching.

c. Lift your arms and bend forward enough so that you can touch the tops of your knees. (If you cannot bend that far, touch as high a point on your legs as you can.)

d. Hold them for a count of five.

e. Repeat steps c and d three more times.

The breathing pattern for this exercise is similar to the pattern in the first stomach exercise:

1. Inhale while checking position.

2. Exhale slowly as you reach for your knees and during the hold.

3. Inhale as you return to lying position.

Lower-back Strengthener

a. Lie on back in same position as for lower-back stretch.

b. Straighten left leg and raise it as high as possible without bending knee.

c. Pull left knee toward you and then straighten it, three to five times. Your leg should pump like a bicycle rider's.

d. Relax leg so that it falls.

e. Repeat *b* through *d* with right leg.

Breathing during the exercise:

1. Inhale as you raise leg.

2. Exhale as you pull knee down.

3. Inhale as you push knee back up.

4. Exhale as you relax leg.

Antipain Exercise

Side stretch

a. Lie on right side.

b. Use a pillow or your arm to support your head and keep neck straight.

c. Bend right leg slightly and let left leg lie behind it.

d. Relax entire body. Let go of all the muscles.

e. Lift your left leg so that the thigh forms a level line with the hip.

f. Slowly bend knee toward the chest. Keep the thigh line level with the hip. You should feel your back stretching.

g. Slide your leg back to the position in step *e*.

h. Hold leg for count of five.

i. Drop left leg behind right. Let entire body go. Wobble a little to loosen the tension.

j. Roll over onto left side and repeat steps *d* through *i*, this time sliding the right leg.

Breathing during this exercise should go as follows:

1. Exhale on *d* as you relax your body.

2. Inhale through nose as you lift your leg.

3. Exhale as you pull your knee forward and slide it back.

4. Inhale as you hold your leg for the count.

5. Exhale as you drop leg and relax body.

These six exercises and the warm-ups should be done every day during the recovery period. It is best if you do them twice a day. The program should continue for three months. Don't expect too much from yourself at the beginning. Write down how you did at the start of the program. You may not want anybody else to know how poorly you fared at the start, but you will enjoy looking at that paper and seeing just how far you have come after three months. Your body should be much more limber after ninety days of flexing.

If you want to do more, that's fine. A stationary bike is a splendid piece of equipment for working out. If you want to get into an exercise program, you should. Be certain, however, that the exercise leader knows about backache. You are not yet ready for exercises that include such back stressors as Marine sit-ups or the yoga plow. Know your own limitations. Some exercises can help some people but may not be right for you. A series of stretching and strengthening exercises known as pilates movements, for example, can do wonders for the back, but they were developed for dancers and assume a very rich body awareness.

If your back flares up again during your recovery, you should set these exercises aside and return to the stretches described for the acute-pain stage. Return to your more demanding exercise program only when you can do those stretches comfortably.

RETURNING TO WORK

Do not expect to work during the acute stage, but once you have firmly settled yourself into the recovery stage you should try to get back to work as soon as possible. This good advice is often difficult to follow. Your union may not let you return to work until you have recovered 100 percent of your ability. Your boss may not want you to come in until you can do more. Employers can be especially reluctant to allow a rehabilitative return in which you are assigned to some less risky labor while your back recovers. If, for example, your old job called for heavy lifting, your employer may not want to put you at a less demanding job. Of course no one with a recovering back should do heavy lifting, so stay home.

Not being permitted to return to work can impede your recovery. Exercise and physical rehabilitation can restore a person's strength, but very few jobs require only strength. You have to recover your skills as well, and rehabilitation cannot give them back. If you work with your hands, get yourself a workbench and a hobby like wood carving. If you work with office machinery, rent a home computer and take the opportunity to upgrade your skills by learning some new piece of software. Whatever you do for a living, if circumstances block your return to work, develop some exercise to sharpen your skills. The union practice of insisting that employees be allowed to stay home to recover fully arose in the days when people who injured their backs were liable to lose their jobs. Well-intended as that policy is, if you hope to work again, get active as soon as possible. You have worked to restore your back. Now work to recover your skills as well.

HELP DURING THE RECOVERY

Once you have put aside the fears of experiencing some dreadful and rare breakdown, you can concentrate on recovering a pain-free life. The number of professionals who are ready and eager to help you is bewildering. There are so many that a patient who hesitates to take charge of the problem can easily go from therapist to therapist for years without seeing one in a duplicate specialty. You can go from chiropractor to acupuncturist to physiotherapist and on and on. To avoid this bouncing from one therapist to another, look for a professional who will teach you how to exercise. You do not want one who simply takes charge while you passively wait to be healed. You need to participate in the healing process. It is not as easy as you might expect to find a practitioner who does not encourage passivity in patients. However, two professionals described in the chapter on acute pain are also notably helpful during the recovery period; these are the physiatrists and kinesiologists.

PHYSICAL THERAPIST. These professionals specialize in muscular problems and can teach exercises to stretch and strengthen specific muscle groups. They are not MDs, and in most states their work still must be prescribed by a doctor. They are considered the most helpful of non-MDs in treating almost any kind of back ailment. To use one ask your GP or orthopedist to prescribe physical therapy. Physical therapists are recommended as the choice for the millions of backache sufferers who do not have access to a physiatrist. Along with exercises, they use many treatments like heat, electrical stimulation, cold, ultrasound, and hydrotherapy that provide temporary relief and comfort. The chief complaint about physical therapists is that they can push a patient too fast. Push yourself but do not ignore pain, and do not let your therapist deny the seriousness of your pain. (In Canada and throughout the British Commonwealth these practitioners are known as physiotherapists.)

OSTEOPATHIC PHYSICIANS. These medical practitioners are licensed to practice in every state. They hold D.O. (Doctor of Osteopathy) degrees instead of M.D.'s and focus on the relationship between muscles and skeletal organization. In addition to using physical manipulation, osteopathic physicians may prescribe drugs and perform surgery. Their techniques often provide immediate relief from acute pain. If you consult an osteopathic physician for chronic back pain, use one who will develop an exercise program for you rather than rely solely on medication and manipulation. (See Chapter Seven for information on back surgery.)

MASSEUR. Massages are usually considered an indulgence because they provide only temporary relief from minor pain; however, it is no indulgence to remind and reassure yourself that pleasure is still possible. And massage can be both pleasurable and relaxing. Full recovery means more than coping with pain. Restore joy to‘your life as soon as you can. You need not use a professional masseur. They seldom have extensive knowledge about backache. Use a wife, husband, or friend. Massages work best in a relaxing environment, and with the application of a lotion or oil. Your partner should work up from feet to waist, waist to neck, and then the scalp. The Japanese massage technique of Shiatsu is not recommended for people with severe backache. This massage concentrates on acupuncture points and is too rough for ordinary backache patients. Especially avoid Shiatsu that includes walking on your back. It is dangerous for anyone with chronic pain to allow someone to walk on the back.

PODIATRIST. One controversial diagnosis of backache is mismatched leg lengths. Your left and right legs should be the same length. If they are not equal, the imbalance can cause back strains. Differences between leg lengths are common but researchers do not agree on the importance of these discrepancies. Some patients, however, do report that they had a wondrous recovery after a podiatrist prescribed a heel lift for a shoe. During your first examination after a back attack, therefore, you should ask your doctor to include a measurement of leg lengths. If a significant discrepancy turns up (greater than one-half inch), consider a podiatrist. Some chiropractors will claim to adjust leg lengths through manipulation, but it is difficult to believe that even very vigorous manipulations can permanently and radically alter such an important skeletal feature.

THERAPIES THAT BRING TEMPORARY RELIEF

Temporary relief is its own reward. Anything that ends discomfort, even for just a short time, is welcome, but temporary relief is not enough to overcome the problem. Relief provides an opportunity to do the activities and exercises that ordinarily hurt too much to pursue.

The spinal manipulations performed by chiropractors, osteopaths, and physical therapists are probably the oldest forms of medical relief for backache. They were controversial 2,500 years ago when Hippocrates invented scientific medicine, and they remain controversial today; however, most patients agree that manipulation, especially in its gentler forms, does relieve moderate back pain for a time. It is not a miracle cure, especially in cases of severe pain. For long-term benefit the manipulation should be part of a program that includes exercise, relaxation, and adaptive activity.

Another popular antipain technique is *hypnosis*, which relaxes the body but does not automatically eliminate or reduce pain. Hypnotism is a method through which a practitioner can suggest perceptions that the subject then experiences. The elimination of pain through hypnosis calls for a negative perception (the absence of a perception) that the hypnotist must specifically and insistently suggest to the subject. Without that suggestion the pain will not disappear. People vary considerably in their susceptibility to hypnosis and it does not work for everyone; however, hypnotizability is an enduring trait, and if you can be hypnotized to see or feel things that are not there, you should be able to hallucinate away pain. Self-hypnosis can also be effective. This technique means you suggest away your own pain. It is best, however, to consult a professional hypnotist first to learn what the suggestive techniques are like and to discover how it feels to be hypnotized.

Acupuncture is an ancient Chinese technique for relieving pain and can often help ease backache. It consists of placing needles in specific parts of the body (known as acupuncture points) to relieve pain in other sites. This method of sticking a pin in point A to ease the pain at point B has given acupuncture a magical quality and the Chinese have developed an elaborate metaphysical explanation for how it works. Western medicine views the traditional Chinese explanation of flows and balances with considerable skepticism but admits that, whatever the explanation, acupuncture frequently causes the temporary relief of pain.

Physiatrists favor a more natural approach and their success in relieving chronic backache makes for a powerful recommendation. Natural techniques of pain relief include water, heat, cold, and movement. These techniques are common to some European spas, but Americans tend to dismiss going to waters for "the cure." Soaking in a bathtub, with or without a whirlpool, is a relaxing way to enjoy the benefits of a spa in your own home.

Technology, too, can offer some help in recovery. One system that has become popular with many doctors is *TENS*, or Transcutaneous Electrical Nerve Stimulation. TENS operates on principles similar to those of acupuncture to excite nerves and overcome pain. Instead of requiring special needles, however, TENS uses a small battery-powered box, about the size of a hand-held remote-control device. The box hooks onto a belt and sends pulses to nerves via electrodes attached to the skin. The basic idea is to jam the painful stimulation by sending strong signals to the affected nerves. This method can provide enough relief to let people do their exercises.

Other technological approaches include *diathermy* and *ultrasound*. Diathermy, like TENS, uses a mild electric current coming from two electrodes. The current heats the soft tissue below the skin. Ultrasound also heats tissue below the skin, but through sonic impulses instead of electricity. These deep-heating techniques once seemed to hold strong promise for pain relief, but are seen now to be no more effective than simpler and less expensive heating devices. Ultrasound has remained more popular with doctors than diathermy and is still used for deep heating. At home the ordinary bathtub soak or old-fashioned hot compress resting against the back works just as well.

FIVE

LIVING WITH A
WELL BACK

Most people do not want to hear that recovering from a painful condition and staying recovered means changing the way they live. Lynn Payer, an authority on how values affect medicine, says in her book *Medicine and Culture* that Americans often favor risky and uncertain operations simply to avoid changing their life-styles. We tend to assume that technology, medication, and surgery can repair whatever is wrong and let us return to our lives as they were before disease struck. But ordinary backache is not a disease that strikes from outside and lays us low. It is a condition that arises from our way of living. An enduring recovery, therefore, requires paying some attention to the problems that brought on the backache. Successful back patients are the ones who change their habits and keep them changed, even after the back pain goes away.

This insistence on lasting change may seem a strange proposition in a book that has accented the goal of reclaiming one's old life. But reclaiming your life does not mean you must restore either the old desperation—the stress that never relaxes—or the old physical imbalances that put your back at risk.

If your work imposes continual tension, you should find ways of shrugging it off when you leave and of slipping moments of relaxation into the work schedule. If your home life is a pressure cooker, look for ways to reduce the anxiety. Many people are reluctant to change their way of living because they do not wish to give up their ambitions. Keep your ambitions but find less destructive ways of satisfying them.

If your work keeps you inactive or exercises only a few of your muscles, you will need to find ways to stretch the other muscles and keep them in shape. That recommendation does not mean you should start jogging five miles a day but walk around the block or, at a minimum, you should become alert enough to notice when your body is too tight. And when your body is tight take action to relax. You should also develop good ways of sitting, standing, and walking. Do not turn off exercising in October and then try to switch it on again in February.

None of these changes require a major shift in your life-style or in your personality. There is no such thing as a "backache personality." In particular, there are no negative personality characteristics that lead to backache. Personality does affect the success of treatment, however. Believing something will work for you can get results. For example, some people are more responsive to placebos than others. (Placebos are treatments that serve no anatomical or physiological purpose.) Some personalities, however, seem to bring more stress into their lives. The so-called Type A personality is more driven than other people, but this need for control does not automatically lead to backache. If relaxing or withdrawing from the pressures of the environment seem difficult, find a simple activity that will allow you to release the tension. A coffee break might be enough to do the trick. Whatever your personality, you need to find ways to balance the stress with relaxation.

Body weight may need to change. Excess weight increases the chances of recurring back trouble. Stretched stomach muscles raise the stress on your lower back by as much as 50 percent. It also changes the direction of stress. The lower back must handle the compression forces exerted by the weight of the upper body pressing down on the spine. A bulging stomach adds a shearing force to the lumbar vertebrae that pulls the spine at right angles from the compressive force. These contrary stresses force the spine in two directions at once, making stability that much harder to maintain. Losing weight is an important way to keep a recovered back healthy.

GOOD POSTURE

Posture refers to the position in which you hold your body. Poor posture places distorting stresses on the spine, and in time the spinal column adapts to these stresses by changing its shape. It is rare for poor posture alone to result in the grotesque spinal curvature one sometimes sees, but poor posture does increase back stress and can make backache more likely. A quick way to check your posture is to stand with your back against a wall. Try to make your back, from shoulders to rump, as flat as you can. Reach behind with a hand and try to slip it between the lower part of your spine and the wall. If the hand goes in easily, you may have a posture problem.

When standing, your weight (center of gravity) should be on the lower vertebrae. To test this weight stand erect and put your fist against your lower back. Now lean forward, rocking out over your feet. You should be able to feel your weight slipping below your fist and running down your legs. If you now rock back, you can feel the weight run up your legs and back. Good posture keeps the weight squarely on your lower back.

When standing, do not hold yourself rigidly to attention or with your knees locked. Keep your back muscles and legs erect but relaxed. If you must stand in one place for a long time, you should get a low footrest. Place one foot on the rest to shift the pelvis and reduce pressure on your spine. People whose work requires long standing in a production line should try to arrange for a footrest at their point of work. Sensible shoes are also important to posture. They should be comfortable and low-heeled.

Posture can also be distorted by carrying a weight for a long time. A heavy bag carried over the shoulder tends to result in uneven shoulders. The bag slips down and the carrier keeps hiking up a shoulder to catch it. Wear the strap across the chest to prevent such a cycle. The introduction of plastic grocery bags is another threat to posture. Their superstrong handles make it easy to carry the bag down at one's side, adding an unbalanced shearing force to the spine. Carry the bag close to the chest or carry two bags, one in each hand, to balance the pulls on your spine.

To improve your posture think of your body as a set of blocks balanced on top of one another. To keep them from slipping and sliding you need to maintain the blocks in a line. Stack the blocks in this manner:

- Lean forward slightly so that your weight is directly over the arches of your feet. If you rock on your feet, keeping your toes and heels still, you will feel the center of your feet. Imagine the blocks of your body centered on a line rising from the arches of your feet.

- Keep your legs straight, but do not lock the knees. Feel the knees over the arches of the feet.

- Now line up the pelvis so that its center is also above the center of your feet.

- The ribs of your chest should be directly above the pelvis.

- With shoulders level, keep head erect so that the neck is clearly visible. Chins that droop hide the neck. Do not tense shoulders; let gravity pull them down.

Practice this posture in the mirror twice a day, but work to develop a sense of yourself so you know how you are standing even when there is no mirror to use. Check your posture from time to time throughout the day—as you stand in line at a store, as you wait for an elevator, while waiting for the DON'T WALK light to change. If it feels strange at first, that sensation is a warning that your body can no longer recognize the proper way to stand. Once you relearn the position you will discover that it is remarkably comfortable. Equally important, good posture is relaxing. Do not feel discouraged if you find that your position is off every time you think to check it. Checking and correcting it relieves stresses that would otherwise continue without rest.

If you find that your posture is unsatisfactory, add the following warm-up exercise to your exercise program. It helps with back flexibility and posture.

a. Sit on floor, legs flat and apart, back erect.

b. Pull your right foot back, placing the heel in your groin and letting the sole of the foot press against the left leg.

c. Raise both arms straight above your head. Try to have the arms and back form a single straight line.

d. Bend forward from the waist and try to grab your left toes with both hands. Keep your back straight.

e. Now curve your back to touch your head to your left knee.

f. Release your toes and *slowly* sit up straight.

g. Straighten out your right leg.

h. Repeat steps *b* through *f*, this time with the left leg tucked.

On step *d* you may find that you cannot reach your toes. Go as far as you can without pain and grab your ankles or calf. You may also find that you cannot put your head to your knee. Bend as far as you can. Breathe as follows:

1. Inhale as you raise your arms.

2. Exhale as you bend forward toward toes. Then inhale as you hold the toes or calf.

3. Exhale as you pull your head down toward your knee.

4. Inhale as you sit back up.

If you feel that your posture is a serious problem, instructors in the *Alexander Technique* may be able to help. Alexander Technique is a system for becoming aware of physical habits. As people learn what they are doing they learn how to stop poor habits and replace them with better ones. The Alexander Technique is not a therapy but a method of instruction. Students, however, often learn ways to improve posture and lessen muscle tension in their backs.

NORMAL ACTIVITIES

Sitting

When seated in a chair you should be able to lean forward, then stand and stretch without pain. A healthy back with healthy disks should be able to endure any of these stresses without a problem. Even so it makes sense to protect your back by using well-designed chairs. Sitting puts much greater stress on the back than standing does, and the kind of sitting found in an office places even more pressure on the back.

Opinion varies as to precisely what makes a "best" chair. In part the answer will depend on your needs. A person working at a keyboard will not want the same chair used by someone relaxing in front of a television. In general a good chair includes these features:

• The *backrest* is the most important detail in a chair. It should be easy to use as you sit in the chair, so the seat itself should not be too deep, especially if you plan to work in it. Some chairs have spring-loaded backrests that follow a person forward. This feature can be a great help if you must lean forward to operate a keyboard, to write, or to observe some detail on a computer monitor. President Kennedy found that rocking chairs let him move forward while keeping his back supported. Canvas backings also allow some flex in the backrest for following a person who leans forward.

- A *pillow* to place between you and the backrest can be a help. In the best of worlds backrests should come down to a point that rests in the normal curve in the lower part of the spine and then angle back. But because we each have our own shape, this curve in a backrest cannot be standardized. Chairs seldom get the back exactly right for any particular individual. A small inflatable pillow can help you adjust to the space.

- *Armrests* significantly reduce the pressure on one's back. Proper armrest placement is important. They should not be so high that you have to hike up your shoulders to use them. Nor should they be so low that you favor one side.

- A *shallow seat pan* does more than make it easy to lean back in the chair. It also gives your legs room to move about. About two thirds of the thigh should be supported. Beyond that the leg, especially the knee area, should be free. You should be able to move your legs freely and stand up easily. You should not be aware of the edges of the chair as you do ordinary work. A seat pan that reaches almost to the knees interferes with that freedom and locks your muscles into a particular position.

- Include a *seat cover* if you find yourself slipping about in the chair. A rough surface helps keep you in place.

- Your feet should touch the floor easily. If the chair is too high, use a *footrest*. You should also use a footrest if you find yourself slumping in your chair. The exhausted slouch in a chair increases lower-back pressure enormously. A low footrest, phone-book size, helps reduce the strain. Another time to use a footrest is when the seat pan is too flat. Our backs do best when we squat instead of sitting regally on a throne. A chair's pan should raise the knees about an inch or so above the base of the buttocks, putting your legs on a slant. If your chair does not slope backward about five degrees, you can create the slant by using a footrest.

As you consider the implications of this list you may realize that many of the chairs in your life have been adding to your stresses. Theater chairs seldom seem to have the right kind of armrests and their cushions may reach all the way to the knees. The sofa in your living room may provide no room at all for your knees to maneuver. The chair at work may have been designed for somebody of quite a different size. "Designer" chairs that present furniture as sculpture are interesting to the eye but hard on the back. Deluxe easy-chairs may be great for lounging, but should not be used if you must get up and down continually. Even your favorite old chair may have been adding stresses to your back.

One especially important chair is the one you sit in while driving a car. Cars put the back at risk even in the best of circumstances, because the steady vibration of engine-powered travel stresses the spine. Pull the driver's seat forward to keep from having to stretch too far and to keep your back against the backrest. The seat belt also helps keep your back against the backrest, and placing a small pillow behind you often increases comfort.

You do not have to change all the chairs you use, but the chair you sit on at work should fit you properly. Take the time to adjust it and find one that fits right. You should also have a chair at home that suits you perfectly. Check it for backrest angle, seat-pan size, and height from floor before you settle on one. If you find that restaurant, movie, and other public chairs do not seem to fit you right, you can carry an inflatable pillow to help adjust the back of any chair to your size.

From time to time a designer claims to have saved the human back by inventing a chair that departs radically from tradition. Chairs that heat the back, vibrating chairs, and chairs that tilt you forward are just a few of the ideas that have been tried. A show-me attitude is usually wisest in these cases. Sometimes the ideas are just plain bad. Mechanical vibration, for example, is not the same as a massage and indeed vibration stresses the back. In other cases the idea may have its specialized uses. A chair that tilts a person forward, for example, can reduce the load on the backs of workers who are half seated, half standing, but most people will find the design odd and gimmicky. A chair that heats the back is another idea that can make sense, but if you really need to heat your back you should be lying down instead of sitting. One radical idea has "sitters" kneel forward. This chair has none of the familiar features—no armrest and no backrest. Instead, "sitters" kneel on a tilted board and knee rests hold them firmly in place. Strange as it seems, the position can be great for short sessions, but is too exhausting for a full day's work.

Sleeping

It is rather startling to learn that there is no real evidence that sleeping on a stiff mattress is actually good for the back. A soft mattress may not be bad for you, but a harder mattress offers one more way to relax the back. More important than the mattress is the sleeping position. Sleeping on one's stomach is the riskiest position. It forces a person to sleep with the head twisted to one side, straining the neck vertebrae and adding tension to the back. In some cases sleeping on the stomach can increase the sway in a person's back. Most people find sleeping on the side best and very comfortable.

Walking

Slightly pigeon-toed walking is a general characteristic of the human species—and for good reason. Imagine a line running on the ground straight ahead of you, passing between your two feet. Normally, a person standing still points the feet at angles of about thirty degrees away from that imaginary line. This position gives good stability, but it adds extra stresses to the muscles when walking. To maintain proper balance we bring our feet toward the imaginary line as we go. (You can see the balance this style gives tightrope walkers.) Bringing the toes slightly inward helps us adapt to the stresses of walking upright. The splayfooted walk, with toes turned outward, stresses the back, legs, and pelvis by forcing the body weight onto the heels instead of over the arches. There are some foot exercises for people whose walk is too splayfooted:

a. Sit on a chair.

b. Raise right foot and flex it, stretching heel toward you and toes out.

c. Return foot to floor in a rocking motion, touching the floor first with the arch, then the ball of the foot, then the toes. Press down with your foot as it touches the floor.

d. Repeat *b* and *c* with left foot.

e. Raise both legs, holding them straight out, with the feet parallel. *Do not allow them to turn out from each other.*

f. Keep heels still and turn toes toward one another. Your goal is to have toes touch one another, although you may find that your feet do not yet have the flex to accomplish that end.

Walking itself is a good exercise for the back. It puts less stress on the back than sitting and it helps one's muscles.

Lifting

Everyone seems to have heard that you should "lift with your legs, not with your back." By that they mean that you should keep your back straight during heavy lifting, bending only the knees. The source of this wisdom is uncertain, but it came into question when occupational researchers noticed how difficult it was to persuade people to keep their backs straight when they lifted. They might bend their legs more, but they tended to bend their backs as well. Computer modeling of the stresses has shown that an erect back is under greater compressive stress than a bent one! Bend your legs and use them to help steady yourself, but bend your back as well to reduce the load on it. The lifting force should, however, come from the legs. Use the whole body.

The best advice about heavy lifting is to do as little of it as possible. It does stress the back and is a major occupational risk for backache. Warm up before doing any serious lifting and make a conscious effort to relax once the task is done. Use some kind of hauling truck or dolly whenever you can.

SPORTS

The idea of the exercises that appear throughout this book is to restore balance to the muscles. Ideally, all the muscles should be able to stretch and flex equally to adapt perfectly to any activity. The out-of-shape couch potato is at risk because so many muscles can barely stretch or flex at all. The athlete who concentrates on only the skills needed to accomplish a particular feat is also at risk because certain muscles will dominate others. Certain sports have a reputation for putting the back more at risk than others, but studies by occupational specialists have found that no particular sport, including tennis, football, and baseball, puts the back at special risk. But some sports do not demand general exercise. Bowling, golf, and some baseball positions are examples. People who limit their exercise to such a sport can hurt themselves because their muscles are too out of balance. An exercise program for preserving a back should include:

• walking,

• swimming,

• the warm-ups described in Chapter 4,

• and the flexibility exercises that follow them.

Runners are famous for wanting to get back into running as quickly as possible, but if a person runs regularly and suffers a back attack, the running part of one's exercise program may have become too dominant. It is easy to persuade couch potatoes that their problem is that they do not exercise enough. It is hard to make them change, but at least they accept the idea that they should be in shape. It is harder to tell runners and other single-minded athletes that they, too, need to exercise better. They already exercise so much. But you can overtrain parts of the body at the expense of other parts. The proof is in the backache.

No one should run during an acute back attack. Wait two or three weeks, at least, before starting again. And if the back attack included sciatic features such as pain extending into the upper leg, you should not run until well into the recovery stage. Walking is a better exercise for the recovering backache sufferer.

If you run, play tennis, bowl, enjoy golf, or engage in any other sport as a regular exercise, keep it up. But do not ignore the rest of your body.

OCCASIONAL TWINGES

Once your back recovers it may be years before it acts up again. If you work at staying healthy, it may never happen again, but the memory of such pain stays with people as a fear. You see the memory in the mattresses people use, in the deliberate way they bend their knees as they pick things up, and in the seriousness with which they view any twinges they do feel. It is right to take those brief pangs and aches seriously. Almost certainly a first back attack was preceded by signs that a more experienced person would recognize as warnings. If you feel your back is beginning to tighten, make a deliberate effort to ease it. Use the emergency knee hug described on page 32. If your back hurts a bit or you strain it, sleeping on the floor for a night or two can help relax it. If you suffer another back attack, do not panic or despair. Take some medication, get into bed for a few days, and put some ice on the sore spot. You survived a back attack before, and will again, although it is hard to be so philosophical when it happens.

HELP AT STAYING WELL

We think of doctors as people to see when we're sick. Checkups are the usual reason for seeing a doctor when you are well. Using doctors to help you stay well is a novel idea. It is a good idea, however, to include professional help in learning how to take full charge of your health.

YOGA TEACHERS. Yoga is an ancient practice that was codified around 500 B.C. It includes a series of posture exercises and breathing techniques that help a person gain control over the body and relax it. Courses in yoga technique can help a person whose backache is well on the way to recovery. Yoga exercises are dangerous during periods of back pain, but are great for eliminating the tensions that can lead to more pain. They keep the muscles stretched and toned.

BIOFEEDBACK INSTRUCTOR. Biofeedback, like yoga, teaches people how to take control of body functions that science calls "involuntary." Classes that teach biofeedback and progressive relaxation techniques offer a proven way of learning how to take control of your body, although they are not so good at muscle toning.

Choosing between yoga and biofeedback seems to be a matter of taste. Do you prefer techniques that are steeped in ancient philosophical tradition or would you rather learn techniques that use the latest technological jargon? However you choose, it is a good idea to learn ways of relaxing during the years ahead.

SIX

CHRONIC PAIN

The pain discussed in this chapter is not typical of most backaches, or even of a large minority of backaches. Overwhelmingly, backache sufferers recover full back function and the pain goes away completely within a few months to half a year after the back attack. Even most of the cases that continue for a longer time are so much improved after six months that a person feels confident that full health is returning. Only a small percentage of back attacks lead to chronic, disabling pain. Yet because the number of backaches is so high, even a small percentage results in a large number of people whose back pain does not seem to go away. It can last for years and take over a person's life. Pain like this is not normal or natural. It indicates that something has gone wrong with the recovery, but it was not until recently that medicine began to understand what must be done to ease the pain.

If your back attack began six months ago and is still a regular nuisance, you need help. If you are still spending much of your time in bed, you need intensive help in treating both your back and the psychological consequences of being disabled by pain for so long.

In recent years special clinics or centers that treat chronic pain have appeared in hospitals around the country. Although people may have chronic pain for many reasons, most of the patients suffer from low-back pain. The centers take a team approach to relieving pain. A typical staff will include a physiatrist, a physical therapist, a psychiatrist, an occupational therapist, a social worker, and a psychologist. They work together to treat the many different ways chronic pain stalls a person's life. The team meets regularly to discuss the individual patients and to coordinate activities. Through these meetings the physical therapist knows what the social worker is hoping to achieve and can direct therapy toward that goal. At the same time the social worker knows what the physical therapist thinks is possible and can help suggest reasonable ambitions for a particular patient.

Part of a pain center's service is an inpatient program that commonly lasts for about three weeks. A group of perhaps eight people will arrive on a single day to begin an intensive program. Some of these patients may have spent the preceding two years in bed. Suddenly they find themselves doing exercises, relaxing in a warm pool, talking to a psychologist, and socializing with other pain sufferers. It is common to hear such patients say that they are exhausted by the end of the day, but they are also proud and encouraged to discover that they can do more than they had hoped possible. It also encourages them to learn that they are not alone in their misery. Pain patients may never have heard of anyone else being as bedridden and uncomfortable as themselves, but during the stay at the center they discover there are other people with the same misery. Many of the patients form a strong sense of identification with the others in the group.

There is no single approach to pain that works for everyone. A critical aspect of each individual's stay at the center is the development of a plan for what the patient will do after leaving the inpatient program. The premise of a pain center's treatment is that by the end of the program each patient should be up and about and not remain dependent on the professionals who are treating them. Plans vary widely. One patient might be a twenty-seven-year-old woman who reacts in absolute horror to the suggestion that she could be disabled for the rest of her life. The plan for her is to restore her to a normal working career. Another patient might be a sixty-year-old man with a similar back injury, but he has done physical labor since school days and is worn out. The plan for him is to get him active again, although it is not expected that he will return to his construction job.

As patients see themselves getting stronger some begin to realize that the causes of their pain extend far beyond the muscles in their backs. It is not unusual to see patients begin to worry that they will relapse as soon as they return to the complications of their home life. The presence of a social worker on the center's team helps the patient and other members of the patient's family begin to wrestle with these larger issues. This concern about home life after the intensive inpatient period is perfectly reasonable. Follow-up studies have shown that patients who are unable to continue working with the pain center on an outpatient basis do not consolidate the gains made during their stay at the hospital. They need continuing help in reclaiming their lives. The importance of remaining as an outpatient with the pain center was made especially clear by surgery statistics. Many pain-program patients have already tried back surgery before coming to the center and are considering further surgery. One study found that 38 percent of those patients who do not continue with the program as outpatients do get repeat surgery. This figure is about the same as in the general population of back-surgery patients. For those patients who do go on to outpatient work, the repeat surgery rate drops to less than 7 percent.

Pain centers are not miracle spas. Slightly more than half of the patients do report a reduced use of medication, an improved ability to cope with pain, and a decrease in the amount of time spent in bed. Yet a little over 20 percent of patients report no improvement as a result of their participation in the program. Chronic pain has not yet been conquered, but the war against it has come a long way. The progress is especially encouraging when we remember how recently the war was declared.

ACUTE vs. CHRONIC PAIN

The growth of pain centers reflects a recent insight: All pain is not alike. Chronic pain differs from acute pain and should not be treated in the same way. Since the days of the Greeks there have been two basic approaches to pain. One is *Stoicism*, also known as the grin-and-bear-it approach. It advises pain sufferers to be brave and to tough it out. Except for brief bouts of acute pain, Stoicism does not work. A stiff upper lip may get you through the anguish of a visit to the emergency room, but Stoicism in the face of chronic pain tends to make people bitter, lonely, and desperate to cling to whatever little compensations life still offers.

The other approach to pain is called *Epicureanism*, or the effort to retain the pleasures of life. This outlook has had a revival as doctors and psychologists have begun to look for practical solutions to chronic pain. The visualization exercises and massage programs recommended in this book reflect this approach. They were specifically designed to help avoid the cycle in which pain's compensations become the only pleasures left in life. Pleasure, of course, is not limited to physical delights. There are emotional and intellectual pleasures as well. Music, hobbies, social interests, and curiosity all provide pleasure. These "pleasures of the soul," as the Greeks called them, seem even more powerful than the pleasures of the body. People can be physically comfortable and yet feel miserable. Meanwhile, others are enduring pain and yet are at peace with themselves and the world because they have cultivated other pleasures. As part of the struggle to end chronic pain, be sure to retain whatever pleasure you can. Stay interested in things; do the visualization exercises; enjoy gentle massages.

If you seek help about chronic pain, find out if your practitioner favors the Stoical or Epicurean approach. Traditional medicine has encouraged Stoicism, and even with the introduction of painkilling drugs doctors still emphasize bravely enduring whatever pain persists. Many doctors see pain as something outside their own specialty. One study of medical textbooks found that out of 22,000 pages, including texts about cancer and surgery, only 54 pages discussed pain. One reason practitioners without M.D.s are so popular among backache sufferers is their tendency to reject Stoicism in favor of more satisfying approaches to pain.

The difference between acute and chronic pain also requires a change in attitude toward painkilling drugs. Medication is important during the acute stage of backache because it lessens pain while the body recovers, and the medication makes a sufferer comfortable enough to do healing exercises. Chronic pain may be temporarily eased by medication, but the body does not improve. Even worse, the medication itself becomes part of the problem.

During the mid-1970s a congressman who had long been famous in Washington for his rectitude and sobriety became embroiled in a national scandal. The incident reached its climax when the congressman appeared on a burlesque stage with a stripteaser. The road to the ruin of his political career began with a chronic backache. In the search for relief he began to drink and the drinking led to other problems. Fortunately for him, he was so well known among Washington insiders as a sobersides that they realized something more than the usual Washington tale of sex and ego had to be afoot. Although he was voted out of office, the former congressman sobered up and was welcomed back to Washington, where he works as a successful lawyer. His story shows that even the most straitlaced of individuals is at risk for addiction when faced with chronic back pain. For many people, recovery from backache must *include* treatment for addiction. I stress the word *include* because, by itself, detoxification will not work. Backache sufferers turn to alcohol and drugs because they do not know what else to do. They need help in overcoming the physical addiction and in finding other ways to deal with their backache. Detoxification is beyond the scope of this book, but if you suffer from chronic back pain, you should stop taking antipain medication. If stopping is difficult, get help fighting the addiction! About a third of the patients who enter the pain center at the Hospital for Joint Diseases in New York need to undergo detoxification for addiction to narcotics.

GETTING UNSTUCK

Another important difference between acute and chronic pain is the goal of treatment. With ordinary backache you want to recover. With chronic backache you want to reach a position from which you can start to recover. Thus many of the practitioners who can help during the acute or recovery stages of a common back attack have little to offer sufferers from chronic pain. Exercise, too, needs to change.

Once a chronic-pain patient gets back on track, the exercises discussed throughout this book should be enough to keep the back fit, but special efforts must be made to restore the body when pain reaches the chronic stage. Find a physical therapist, a physiatrist, or a kinesiologist who will work with you to improve your conditioning, increase your body's flexibility, and relax any tight muscles. You know you have found a good one if your receive clear guidance on how to help yourself.

Chronic-pain victims are almost always in poor physical shape. They spend too much time in bed and allow their cardiovascular systems to degenerate. To restore some measure of fitness they should walk, work on a stationary bike, and climb stairs. Walking around the block may be all a person can do. Take that level as the starting point and then build on it. Walk around the block each day and add a hundred yards to each third journey. After three days such a person can walk around the block, go fifty yards beyond the home, and then walk back to the entrance. After two weeks of this exercise a person has added another lap around the block to the effort.

Chronic-pain sufferers should also work at those everyday tasks that give them trouble. If ordinary chores like climbing stairs, making the bed, or sitting in a chair are hard, practice them. Stretch exercises, like those described in Chapter 3, are also good practice for chronic-pain victims. If stretching seems difficult, take a warm bath and do the exercises while relaxing in the tub.

BEHAVIORAL CHANGES

Chronic-pain victims often know people who scoff at their pain and who accuse the sufferer of malingering or of being a bit crazy. People in pain, of course, know very well that they really do hurt and they often become defensive and resentful at any suggestion that their pain may include a psychological side. Yet it is virtually impossible to be in pain for months without having the pain affect one's attitude and behavior. Here is a simple self-examination to see where you stand:

Attitude Toward Pain

1. *Are you preoccupied by thoughts of pain?* You may feel that the correct answer is "No more than reasonable, given my circumstances," but that natural pre-

occupation is the point. This question asks if pain is blinding you to your own life. Do you find that because of the pain you often lose track of time or of the lives of friends and family?

YES _____ NO _____

2. *Do you find it hard to enjoy even the best moments?* Does the knowledge that pain lurks behind every corner enter your thoughts and affect your actions even when pain is temporarily absent?

YES _____ NO _____

3. *Has the pain made you realize some gloomy "truths" about yourself?* Do you see yourself more pessimistically now? Do you expect failure? Do you feel guilty or ashamed for having let yourself down?

YES _____ NO _____

4. *Have you discovered any secret satisfactions in chronic pain?* For instance, in the last question, did you find that you said to yourself "Of course I am a failure, but it is the pain's fault, not mine." And did that explanation seem comforting? Do you find that pain excuses (in your own mind) the many inadequacies that are part of everyday life? Does it let you get your way with family members who might not otherwise be so pliable?

YES _____ NO _____

Changes in Life-style

5. *Do you depend on medication* or other forms of pain deadeners, including alcohol, to get you through the day?

YES_____ NO _____

6. *Do you seek out new doctors,* going from one to another in search of that special healer who can help you?

YES _____ NO _____

7. *Has your social life declined?* Have you stopped visiting and telephoning friends? Have they, for whatever reason, fair or unfair, stopped calling?

   YES _____   NO _____

8. *Has your sex life stopped?*

   YES _____   NO _____

9. *Is your temper harder to control?*

   YES _____   NO _____

10. *Have you grown more dependent on family members?* Do you feel you can stand up to them less than you once did because you depend so much on them for help?

    YES _____   NO _____

If you answered "Yes" to two or more questions in each part of this little examination, pain appears to be affecting your behavior. You are NOT going crazy, not showing signs of Freudian neurosis, and—most of all—this does not mean the pain is "just in your head." But pain erodes the soul as well as the body, and most sufferers need counseling in order to get back on their feet and regain control over their lives.

For example, chronic-backache sufferers are out of action so much that often they can no longer organize their lives enough to do the things they need to get done. The diary activities recommended in earlier chapters were geared at avoiding this trap by encouraging readers to see right from the start what the backache was doing to their lives. Chronic-backache sufferers often need to relearn basic time-management skills.

Another common problem associated with the enforced idleness of chronic pain is an altered sense of oneself. Chronic-backache victims can forget they have needs beyond simply reducing their pain. Victims can make a kind of loser's pact with those people on whom they depend. Without ever saying the words aloud, they agree to make no other personal demands if the limitations imposed by their pain are accepted. So they lie in bed or watch what others watch on television, contributing little and getting less from life. They need to relearn all the other things there are in living. They must rediscover the importance of personal time, of getting out of the home for personal pleasure and social companionship.

WHAT IS CHRONIC PAIN AND WHY DO YOU FEEL IT?

Pain is one of medicine's and psychology's deepest mysteries. It is entirely subjective, felt only by the victim, and yet the victim knows it as one of the most basic truths of existence. Everyone is familiar with acute pain. It can be sharp and disabling, but it rapidly reaches a crisis. Then it begins to fade, although it may not disappear immediately. A typical example of acute pain follows a hammer blow to a finger that holds a nail. The pain is sudden and intense, but soon disappears. Indeed the pain may be gone long before the finger loses its black-and-blue color.

Back attacks begin with acute pain, meaning, in medical terms, that the crisis comes quickly. The pain should then gradually subside. It takes longer to recover from a back attack than to get over a hammer blow to the finger, but most people will find that the exercises, techniques, and medical attention discussed in previous chapters can restore them quickly to an active pain-free life.

Then there is pain that does not go away. Its intensity varies, but time does not heal it. Many people's instinct is to treat chronic pain the same way they treat acute pain, with rest and medication, but chronic pain is not simply acute pain dragged out over time. Something is keeping the pain from fading. Besides its physical and psychological aspects, chronic pain usually develops a large social component as it sucks most of a person's life into its black hole. Everything becomes involved in chronic pain—a person's family life, marital life, and work life. Treatment of chronic backache demands attention to the whole person.

When it comes to treatment, medicine has been more successful at finding practical techniques that can relieve acute pain. That victory began more than a century ago when anesthesia was introduced into surgery. Painkilling medication quickly followed. This success inspired fairly simple mechanical models of what pain is and how to treat it. One old theory saw pain as a kind of push-button reaction. Theorists proposed the notion of "pain nerves," which worked like other sensory nerves. Textbooks used to say there were pain nerves just below the skin in the same way that the skin has nerves that respond to heat or to pressure. Trigger such a nerve, doctors speculated, and you feel pain. If the theory were correct, all one would have to do to conquer pain would be to prevent the signal from reaching the brain. It turns out, however, that there are no such pain nerves and the old push-button idea is wrong.

Today's dominant theory of acute pain is called the gate-control theory, proposed in 1965 by Ronald Melzack and Patrick Wall. Its basic idea is that the nervous system processes a variety of sensory stimulations and, under certain conditions, allows the stimuli to become pain. The theory sees the processing point as a gate that keeps most stimulation from continuing onward, but sometimes the gate does open and a person experiences pain. That theory suggests that you could treat pain by shutting the gate and locking it for a time.

The gate and push-button theories see pain as something out there to be thwarted, and to a fair extent that vision has worked well with acute pain. Anesthetics and narcotics allow surgeons to perform wonders. Analgesic medication sold over the counter has made pain relief a part of everyday life. Naturally people have come to think of pain as a kind of demon that can be exorcised by taking the right chemicals. So, of course, when backache begins people look for the right medication that can relieve the pain and let them go on with their business.

This understanding of pain collapses when we consider chronic pain. Neither narcotics nor bedrest can overcome persistent physical misery. Chronic ache shows us that rather than being an invading demon, pain is a subjective perception of one's own body. As such it is affected by much more than a hurtful event, and there is no simple correlation between the amount of pain and the amount of physical damage done. For one thing, different people are susceptible to different levels of pain. We do not know why. Mood, self-respect, ambition, happiness, and body image all play a part. If a person feels happy and healthy, a sudden ache will seem like an intrusion. The pain inspires a person to act to end the ache, but does not challenge that basic view of oneself as healthy. If a person is anxious and does not feel healthy, pain seems sharper and more distressing. You can observe this simple biological fact by watching two dogs fight. During the row both seem oblivious to pain, but when one begins to flee it is likely to yip in agony if the victor so much as swipes at it. Anxiety and fear amplify pain. Backache poses a special risk for fear-induced pain because an acute attack does take a fairly long time to heal. During that period a person's self-image may change. Instead of thinking of oneself as basically healthy, the sufferer thinks, "I am a person who hurts." That change in attitude can alter the effects of the pain as well. We begin to yip at twinges.

Pain for this person is nothing like acute pain in the normal victim of a back attack. Now the idea of pain as an alien demon becomes more of a hindrance than a help. It encourages people to seek partial solutions to an elaborate problem. They continue to hunt for *the* drug or *the* therapeutic technique that will block the pain. Second, the notion of pain as an outside force blinds people to what their lives are becoming as pain leaves a person unable to work, uninterested in food, and generally depressed.

Yet even for chronic pain recent medical news has gotten much better. By combining physical therapy with counseling to overcome the psychological erosions of pain, patients who once seemed doomed to a life of disability are getting back on the road to recovery.

SEVEN

SURGERY AND OTHER DESPERATE MEASURES

In a small number of back attacks a physical problem blocks the road to recovery. Usually the blockage comes from a disk that has ruptured so badly that fragments from inside the disk have spattered against ligaments and nerve. In these cases surgery provides the surest and quickest relief. The fragments pose the same kind of problem that a splinter in the finger raises. You cannot truly recover until the splinter is out. A surgical procedure developed in the 1930s can provide the same sort of instant relief your mother used to give when she got a sliver out from your hand. Of course the back is not the hand and full recovery takes a bit longer, but removal of the disk fragments sets the patient on the road to normal development.

Surgery is preferable to other techniques for getting rid of disk fragments. One procedure that had a brief popularity was chemonucleolysis, the use of a chemical to dissolve part of the disk. The chemical favored is chymopapain, an extract from the papaya fruit. If successful, it is cheaper and quicker than surgery. The entire procedure takes no more than half an hour. The procedure's greatest problem has been the number of unpredictable bad reactions. About a third of the patients develop excruciating pain that can last as long as two days. One percent of patients have an allergic reaction; in a few cases the reaction is fatal. Enthusiasts of the chymopapain injection liked to say it is "seventy-five percent effective where bedrest and traction failed." That statistic (based on Food and Drug Administration tests) ignores the point that when bedrest fails, there is almost always some real impediment to recovery—a psychological, social, or physical block. The more serious question is how it does when compared to other efforts to remove whatever is blocking recovery. If the block is psychological, studies indicate that chymopapain is no better than any other placebo. When the problem is physical, chymopapain can do the trick. The allergic risk seems excessive, however, since there is an alternative and since the disk fragments themselves are not life-threatening. If your doctor recommends this approach, be sure that you are fully tested for allergic risks before consenting to the procedure.

For all its utility, surgery to treat a ruptured disk has acquired something of a poor name in the world of backache. It is performed far too often. Even if your doctor tells you directly that you have a ruptured or degenerated disk and need surgery, chances are high that you do not. One survey of backache patients found that 75 percent of those who had been told that they needed surgery recovered without getting it. Remember that the point of this surgery is to unblock an impeded recovery. Disk surgery, therefore, is difficult to justify until patients and doctors alike know that the recovery process is stuck. Even then you must be sure that the reason for the blockage is physical. Problems with your job or home life are not going to be cured on the operating table.

If you see a doctor about an acute backache and receive a recommendation for immediate surgery, ask many questions. Why the hurry? Is there no hope that bedrest, ice, and exercise will do the trick? Is yours a special case or does this doctor routinely recommend surgery? What is the purpose of the operation? Is it to accomplish something specific or is it to explore the problem more fully? What kind of rehabilitation program will you need and receive? You may get good answers. If you received a serious blow to the back or if CAT scan imaging shows clear disk fragments, there may be no point in waiting. Usually, however, you should wait at least two months to see how your back does on its own. Don't make that two months of bed rest. Try to do the stretches, exercises, and other procedures described in earlier chapters.

The diagnosis of a ruptured disk with fragments calling for surgery usually comes in two steps. Part one: The examining practitioner sees that the pain is abnormally severe and remote. If, for example, a touch to the foot or calf brings cries of agony, the examining professional knows that this degree and spread of pain is usually associated with a ruptured disk. Part two: imaging. This step is new. Formerly, there was no way to confirm the diagnosis until the patient was on the operating table because disk fragments do not appear in X rays, but modern imaging systems like computerized tomography (CAT) and magnetic resonance imaging (MRI) do show the fragments. The ability to detect fragments before the operation means that so-called exploratory surgery is less justified than ever.

If fragments are discovered, competent physiatrists and kinesiologists will both refer you to surgeons. The surgeon, however, is only a detour. Once a diskectomy—as the surgical removal of a herniated disk is known—has been performed, you will need a good rehabilitation program. Discuss this postoperative therapy both with the practitioner who recommends seeing a surgeon and with the surgeon. Arrange for a rehabilitative program before going into surgery.

Before agreeing to back surgery it is also good to get a second opinion. If experts agree that surgery is necessary *and* agree on the diagnosis, take their opinion seriously. It is a bad idea to agree to back surgery if the diagnosis is vague. The one common risk of a diskectomy comes from the inevitable formation of scar tissue. Normally the scar does not lead to problems, but sometimes it does. The reasons are unknown and the risk in any particular case cannot be predicted.

Do not spend the presurgical period in bed. Act as though you were suffering a normal acute back attack and follow the recommendations given in Chapter 3. Walking around does not hurt the disk. Do the exercises that you can muster and follow the other parts of the program, such as visualization, keeping a diary, and shoulder shrugging.

The procedure itself is relatively straightforward. Hospitalization generally lasts three or four days. The recovery period following the return from the hospital typically lasts three to four weeks. Look on this period as a time following an acute back attack and follow the program described in the chapter on acute backache. One difference, however, is help. Do not try to recover on your own. No matter how fine you feel, use a physiatrist, physical therapist, or kinesiologist to help you recover.

After a month you should be sufficiently recovered to return to work. The program in the chapter on the recovery stage presents the outlines of exercises and recovery for this period, but, again, use a professional to guide your rehabilitation. Six months after the operation you should have fully recovered, leaving the surgery a distant memory.

From one third to 40 percent of all back surgery fails. That disturbing figure misleads a bit, however, because not all spinal surgery is performed to remove disk fragments. Some other reasons for surgery are:

- *lumbar stenosis,* or narrowing of the spinal cord's canal in the vertebrae of the lower back. Stenosis is one of those deviants from the ideal spinal form that may cause no problem at all. This surgery is justified only if the backache includes pain below the knee and images of the spine show a clear abnormality.

• *terrible pain.* Sometimes when the pain seems unendur-
able surgeons try to intervene. An operation known as
rhizotomy seeks to end the pain by cutting nerves in
the spinal cord. The technique was developed as an
experiment and has mostly failed. Another antipain
procedure is a nerve-block injection. It uses a steroid or
alcohol to numb the nerves around the painful area. It
can work or do harm, depending on the expertise of the
doctor. Find out about your doctor's past attempts and
successes before agreeing to this procedure.

• *spinal instability.* Orthopedic surgeons sometimes join
two disks together. This fusion has a certain prestige
since it has been performed on some famous athletes;
however, it is performed too often. The fusion itself
creates a stiff spot in the back. Above that point the
back may become even more unstable, swinging like a
stick on a pivot. Less common, but also seen, is a new
instability below the fusion. Sometimes fusion patients
are told they will need another operation to fuse the
disks above or below the previous operation. Rather
than helping, the effect of repeated fusions may be like
having one's back zippered shut.

• *scoliosis,* or a severe curving of the spine to the side.
This condition has no connection with the common
back attack and is an important candidate for surgery,
especially during a person's childhood.

Back surgery is performed by both orthopedic surgeons
and neurosurgeons. For surgery associated with common
back attacks neurosurgeons have a somewhat better
reputation among back patients, although it is difficult
to find medical professionals who are willing to go on
the record concerning this delicate matter. Dr. Williband
Nagler, physiatrist and chief of the rehabilitation depart-
ment at New York Hospital, did second the judgment.
"This is just a matter of opinion, not science," he said,

"but neurosurgeons are doubly-doubly careful about not doing any damage to the nerves. Orthopedic surgeons like to get the back as straight as possible, and that is less important."

EIGHT

A READY REFERENCE
TO BACKACHE

The material in this section can be used in two ways. First, it is a dictionary for quickly checking a point raised elsewhere in the book. A more important use is to provide specific information that has not been appropriate for the general discussion. For example, there are a number of relatively rare back disorders, and one of them may be applicable to you. Many of these problems are listed here so that, if you need to know a particular term, you can find it.

This ready reference combines two types of listing. First, it is an ordinary dictionary, with all words listed in alphabetical order. Second, it contains six specialized glossaries about the back. One glossary lists terms relating to the back's anatomy. These entries are preceded by the letter A. Here you will find the names of bones, ligaments, and other parts of the body that make up the back. A second glossary lists medical conditions that can strike the back—look for the letter C. A third, preceded by the letter T, lists therapies used in treating the back. The fourth glossary names some common medications used by backache patients—look for the letter M. The fifth, next to the letter P, lists practitioners of various sorts who can treat the back. The final glossary lists terms that fall under none of the other categories. If, for example, you want to know more about the medication used in backache treatment, just scan the glossary. Wherever you spot an *M* you know the word to the right falls into the medication glossary. If you want to know about doctors and others who can help with backache, scan the glossary for the letter *P*. This system lets a reader find related definitions. At the same time it lets a person check the meaning of a particular backache term simply by looking up the word in its alphabetical position.

anatomy
  conditions
    therapies
      medication
        practitioner
          other

M *acetaminophen*: the active ingredient in Tylenol; an analgesic medication.

O *acute backache*: pain in the back that quickly reaches a crisis (see Chapter 3). It contrasts with chronic backache.

C *adhesion*: fibers that form within joints to connect tissues that are normally separate. They can be a source of back pain and can limit movement.

C *adolescent kyphosis*: excessive curvature of the back. Often called Scheuermann's disease, it is most readily diagnosed and treated in teenagers.

T *Alexander Technique*: a system for developing conscious control over physical habits. Instructors can be helpful in developing good posture.

anatomy
| conditions
| | therapies
| | | medication
| | | | practitioner
| | | | | other

M   *analgesic*: a painkilling medication.

C   *ankylosing spondylitis*: progressive stiffening of the spine; an inflammatory disease far more common in men than in women. Its severe form can force a person to bend forward, facing the ground, while walking.

A   *annulus fibrosus*: the outermost part of the spinal disk. It surrounds the nucleus pulposus (see) the way a tire tread protects an inner tube. It is constructed like a radial tire, with strong fibers around it to keep the disk stable and the joints of the vertebrae secure. Although its fibers are stronger than steel, it can sometimes develop a bulge or even burst.

A   *apophyseal joints*: the joints along both sides of the vertebrae. They make the spine flexible, supporting both compression forces from above and shearing forces from the side.

C   *arachnoiditis*: an inflammation of the connective tissues surrounding the spinal cord. It is a risk of myelography (see).

C   *arthritis*: inflammation of a joint. Arthritis in many joints, by limiting motion, can add to back stress.

T   *arthrodesis*: a surgical procedure, sometimes performed on the spine, to relieve pain by fusing a joint.

anatomy
| conditions
| | therapies
| | | medication
| | | | practitioner
| | | | | other

M   *aspirin*: a common analgesic for moderate backache. It seems to work on peripheral nerves rather than on the brain itself. Although it has some side effects, they are usually less severe than those of many prescription drugs and it is, therefore, popular for backaches.

O   *Babinski's test*: a test for brain or spinal disease. It checks for the response of toes to scratching on the sole of the foot. The toes of a patient with a healthy spinal cord will flex downward; those of a patient with a diseased upper spine will fan apart and the big toe will move up.

T   *behavioral analysis*: recording how one passes the time. The diary technique advocated in this book is a simple example. Chronic backache sufferers are often startled to realize how limited their live's have become.

T   *biofeedback*: a technique for learning how to relax and gain conscious control of the body. However it is learned, the ability to relax is an important part of maintaining a healthy back.

O   *braces*: physical supports worn on the body. They commonly provide some relief during acute backache, but if worn too much can retard recovery.

anatomy
   conditions
      therapies
         medication
            practitioner
               | other

C   *brucellosis*: a bacterial infection that can cause spinal disease. It is a risk of unpasteurized milk. It is very rare in the United States.

C   *bursitis*: an inflammation of a bursa, or lubricating saclike structure, within a joint. It can limit motion and lead to stresses on the back.

A   *cervical spine*: the neck. It consists of seven vertebrae and is the most mobile part of the spine, allowing great motion in turning the head. After the lumbar spine it is the most likely region for backache.

T   *chemonucleolysis*: a procedure for dissolving portions of a spinal disk by injecting a chemical into it (See chymopapain).

P   *chiropractor*: a practitioner trained in spinal manipulation techniques developed by R. R. Palmer. Their method is controversial and intensely disapproved of by many medical doctors, but they treat far more backache patients than do doctors. For lasting relief most backache patients will need more than manipulation (see entry on kinesiologist). During severe pain gentle manipulations are preferable to the more forceful ones of traditional chiropractics.

anatomy
   conditions
      therapies
         medication
            practitioner
               other

C   *chronic backache*: pain in the back that time does not seem to heal properly. Although only a small minority of backaches become chronic, the damage it takes on human happiness and economic productivity each year is very high.

T   *chymopapain*: extract from the papaya fruit sometimes used to dissolve the ruptured gel from a damaged disk (see chemonucleolysis). Because of the risk of a serious or even fatal allergic reaction, this technique is not recommended. When it does work the relief from sciatic pain in the leg is almost immediate.

C   *coccydynia* or *coccygodynia*: pain in the tailbone, commonly caused by a bruise received during a fall.

A   *coccyx*: the tailbone. It consists of four small vertebrae fused into one bone. Although it can be bruised from a fall, it is seldom part of a common backache.

O   *computerized axial tomography* (CAT): an imaging process for interpreting X rays. A computer processes an X ray to provide sectional pictures of the body. It is sometimes used in checking for disk problems that normally would not appear in an X ray. CAT scans can detect the free fragments from a truly herniated disk.

anatomy
   conditions
      therapies
         medication
            practitioner
               other

T   *cordotomy*: surgical cutting of pain pathways in the upper portion of the spinal cord. It is a last-resort method of relieving pain in patients with cancer. It does not slow the cancer's growth or ease the mental distress of being so ill, but it does reduce the pain caused by the cancer.

M   *Darvon*: a common analgesic for moderate backache.

M   *Demerol*: a common analgesic for moderate to severe backache.

T   *diathermy*: a technique for generating heat below the skin by the use of an electric current. Simpler methods of producing heat are thought to be just as effective.

M   *diazepam*: a commonly prescribed antitension medication. Although it is not a painkiller, it is sometimes prescribed for anxiety-related pain; the active ingredient of Valium.

A   *disk*: a gelatinous, thin tissue found between each of the vertebrae. It keeps the bones from rubbing against one another and provides maneuverability in the joints. It is mostly water (80 percent) and is composed of the annulus fibrosus (see) and the nucleus pulposus (see). The disks are subject to natural aging. They lose water and

anatomy
   conditions
     therapies
       medication
         practitioner
           other

grow thinner, causing the spine to shrink, so that older people are less tall than in their youth. Under stress a disk can bulge or burst.

T   *diskectomy*: the surgical removal of a herniated disk.

M   *DMSO*: a controversial painkiller. Because of its side effects it is illegal to use it for soft-tissue injury (the major cause of backache) or arthritis pain.

C   *duodenal ulcer*: an inflammation or lesion of the entry to the small intestine. Backache can be an important symptom.

A   *dura mater*: a *tough* protective membrane that surrounds the spinal cord. It is extremely sensitive to pain and may start to ache if part of the back (like a ruptured-disk fragment) presses on it.

O *electromyogram (EMG)*: a test to determine if a problem of movement lies in the muscle or in the nervous system.

O *endorphins*: natural painkilling chemicals released in the brain. The most effective backache treatments during the recovery period seem to be those that encourage the natural development of endorphins. Techniques that rely on artificial pain relief, as in drugs, seem to do less well.

anatomy
| conditions
| | therapies
| | | medication
| | | | practitioner
| | | | other

O *Epicureanism*: an approach to pain that strives to keep physical pleasure and joyful emotion in one's life. Contrast it with Stoicism.

A *epidural space*: the space between the dura matter and the vertebrae. It is the site for some injections into the back.

O *ergonomics*: the study of the relation between people and their working environment. It can be important in developing work sites that reduce stress on the back.

T *facet rhizotomy*: see rhizotomy.

C *facet syndrome*: pain in the apophyseal joints (see).

A *femoral nerve*: a nerve sometimes involved in backache. Pain shoots into the groin and upper leg, but not below the knee.

C *fibrositis*: old-fashioned diagnosis for nonspecific aching of the back.

O *functional pain*: a vague term for pain that impedes activity but cannot be explained and does not go away.

O *gate-control theory*: a theory of pain put forward in 1965 by Ronald Melzack and Patrick Wall. It proposes that within the spinal cord there is a "gate mechanism" that opens and closes in response to pat-

anatomy
  conditions
    therapies
      medication
        practitioner
          other

terns of neural stimulation. An open gate leads to pain. Although at present it is the dominant theory of pain, it can mislead backache sufferers into ignoring or downplaying the importance of exercise, emotion, and natural healing to their recovery.

O *Harrington rods*: metal rods used to stabilize the spine in the area of a fracture. They are sometimes used after surgery, especially for when treating scoliosis.

C *herniated disk*: a spinal disk that protrudes beyond its normal range.

T *hypnotism*: a method of suggesting experiences. It can be used to reduce pain if the hypnotist insists forcefully that the pain is gone.

C *iatrogenic*: brought on by medical treatment. An iatrogenic condition is one that arose because of a doctor's words or actions. Chronic backache is sometimes iatrogenic. A patient who is discouraged from exercise and encouraged to wait another week to see if the suffering subsides is at risk for iatrogenic chronic pain.

A *iliolumbar ligaments*: sturdy ligaments connecting the lowest lumbar vertebrae to the pelvis; a common site of back strain.

anatomy
   conditions
      therapies
         medication
            practitioner
               other

A   *interspinous ligaments*: ligaments that extend from the bony knob of one vertebra to the bony knob of the next vertebra. They can tear during sudden severe blows that arch the spine, producing pain that can last for a long time.

A   *intertransverse ligaments*: ligaments that extend from the bony knob on one side of a vertebra to the bony knob on the other side of the same vertebra. They keep a person from leaning too far to one side.

A   *intervertebral foramina*: openings through which spinal nerves leave the spinal column. They provide a vulnerable point where disks and joints can press on a nerve if something goes wrong.

    P   *kinesiologist*: a chiropractor who has been further trained in the mechanics and anatomy of movement. Their extra training gives them an advantage over regular chiropractors in the treatment of backache.

  C   *kyphosis*: a curvature of the spine that bends a person forward; often called a "widow's hump."

   T   *laminectomy*: surgery to remove a part of the vertebra adjacent to a disk. Its usual purpose is to reduce pressure on the spinal cord and the nerves emerging from it.

anatomy
  | conditions
  | | therapies
  | | | medication
  | | | | practitioner
  | | | | | other

A   *ligament*: fibrous connective tissue. The back uses many ligaments to support and stabilize the spine. They can tear or sprain, resulting in baffling, long-lasting pain. The ligaments bear the main stretching loads of the back.

C   *locked back*: popular term for a sudden, painful immobility of the back. It often bends a person into strange shapes. The causes are mechanical, and alarming as the condition is, it does not arise from a sudden disease.

A   *longitudinal ligaments*: the two long ligaments that trace the length of the spine from its top down to the sacrum. They provide stability along the entire spinal column.

C   *lordosis*: the forward curve of the lower spine. Some lordosis is natural for a spine, but too great a lordosis can increase stress on the back.

C   *lumbago*: an old term for any pain in the lower back that does not extend down the legs; lower backache.

T   *lumbar puncture*: a painful procedure known commonly as a "spinal tap." A sample of fluid is taken from the spinal column for further study. It is not done lightly and is not a routine part of a back examination.

anatomy
  conditions
    therapies
      medication
        practitioner
          other

C   *lumbar stenosis*: a narrowing of the spinal canal in the lower vertebrae. Normal variability in human bodies raises great difficulty in judging stenosis. Canals and other openings can be measured, but there is no clear relation between size and risk for backache.

C   *lumbar strain*: another term for unexplained backache. Usually indicates that the problem arises from a muscular strain.

A   *lumbar vertebrae*: the lower-back spine. It is composed of five vertebrae, the broadest and heaviest bones in the spine. They bear the compressive load of the back and are the most likely site of the damage that produces backache.

    T   *McKenzie exercises*: a system of exercises that promotes extension of the back instead of forward flexion. Many patients find them helpful.

      M   *magnesium salicylate*: the active ingredient in popular backache medication such as Doan's pills. It can relieve aching muscles.

        O *magnetic resonance imaging* (MRI; also called NMR, nuclear magnetic resonance): an imaging process that is becoming more popular than CAT scans; it offers longitudinal scanning and does not use radiation.

anatomy
 | conditions
 | | therapies
 | | | medication
 | | | | practitioner
 | | | | | other

T   *Maitland exercises*: a system of manipulations often used by physical therapists to make the spine more flexible.

T   *manipulation*: the movement of bones and other body organs by a trained practitioner. It is often a noisy operation, as the joints release gases during their movement. It can bring temporary relief for backache, but should not be accepted as the only treatment for your back. Gentle manipulation is preferable during backache and manipulation during an acute back attack is inadvisable. Many physical therapists prefer the term "joint mobilization" for a similar therapy.

T   *medcolator*: an electronic device for stimulating the muscle toward exhaustion. It is used to help relax extremely tight muscle spasms.

T   *meditation*: an example of programmed relaxation; the ability to relax at will. Backache is the frequent companion of unrelieved stress, and meditation is a good way of relaxing the body.

M   *methyl salicylate*: the active ingredient in popular backache rubs such as Ben-Gay and InfraRub. It can offer temporary relief and the application of the rub is often comforting.

anatomy
  conditions
    therapies
      medication
        practitioner
          other

T   *mobilization*: see manipulation.

    O *myelography*: a technique for injecting a special dye into the spinal canal so that disk protrusions or tumors can be detected by X ray. This technique should be done only in the face of a most compelling reason. Raise the question of arachnoiditis (see) with your doctor before agreeing to the procedure.

C   *myeloma*: cancer of the bone marrow. Its onset is often painless.

C   *myoligamentous lumbar-sacral strain*: low-back pain.

C   *myositis*: low-back pain. Literally it means an inflammation of the muscles.

A   *neural canal*: the tunnel through the spine through which passes the spinal cord. Also known as the spinal canal and vertebral canal.

    P *neurologist*: a medical doctor specializing in the nervous system. A good source for a second opinion concerning any proposed surgery or concern over nerve damage.

A   *nucleus pulposus*: the inner part of a disk; made of a jellylike material. Under pressure it does not compress but bulges, and if pressed too much, will burst through the annulus fibrosus (see).

anatomy
   conditions
      therapies
         medication
            practitioner
               | other

O *organic pain*: a vague term for pain that seems to have some discernible cause or which goes away and does not become chronic.

P *orthopedist*: a medical doctor who specializes in diseases of the skeletal system. Most backache does not arise from bone problems and is beyond the range of a typical orthopedist. The many rare diseases of the spine that do lie within orthopedic competence can, however, be treated by no one else.

O *orthotic*: an insert for the shoe that alters posture and leg length for cases of backache arising from mismatched leg lengths. Also known as arch supports, lifts, and shoe inserts.

C *osteoarthritis*: degenerative joint disease arising from wear and tear. Also known as "old age arthritis." The lower back is vulnerable to it because of the years of pressure and movement that wear down the cartilage protecting the surfaces of the joints between the vertebrae.

C *osteomalacia*: an abnormal softening of bone. It generally reflects a deficiency in vitamin D, calcium, and phosphorus.

T *osteopathy*: a system of manipulative treatment. Its emphasis on medication and manipulation without attention to teaching the

anatomy
| conditions
| | therapies
| | | medication
| | | | practitioner
| | | | | other

   patient what to do means that in many cases it has only limited success. Osteopaths have a reputation for being willing to treat cases of chronic pain that everyone else has given up on.

A   *osteophytes*: bony spurs.

C   *osteoporosis*: a weakening of the bone as it loses some of its density. Although the bones of both men and women older than age forty begin to lose bone mineral, severe weakening of the bone is more common in older women than in men.

C   *Paget's disease*: painful enlargement and abnormality of bones. It often strikes the lower spine; it is rare in people under forty.

A   *pelvis*: the bony girdle that shapes the hips. It lies below the lower spine and must be highly flexible. It works wondrously well as the body's center of gravity, but from time to time it contributes to backache.

O   *perception*: the experience that makes raw sensory stimulation meaningful. It occurs in the higher brain centers and depends on past learning. It is also affected by mood, ambition, and attitude. Thus, two people with very similar sensory stimulation may have widely differing perceptions. Although perception is always mysterious, the per-

anatomy
| conditions
| | therapies
| | | medication
| | | | practitioner
| | | | | other

ception of backache pain is even more baffling than usual because the nature of the sensory stimulation is often uncertain. Treatment of chronic backache pain should include treatment of all aspects of a person's life that affect perception, including those elements that are not part of the sensory stimulation.

M   *Percodan*: a common analgesic for moderate to severe backache.

P   *physiatrist*: a medical doctor who specializes in physical and rehabilitative medicine. Physiatrists emphasize natural healing methods, issues of life-style, and stress as well as physical aspects of the body. Recommended as the most helpful medical doctor able to treat backache.

P   *physical therapist*: a specialist in developing exercises and programs to rehabilitate the body. They are recommended as the most able of nonmedical doctors for treating back pains. In most states their patients must be referred to them by a doctor, but the trend is toward direct access. In other countries these practitioners are sometimes known as physiotherapists.

C   *pinched nerve*: a common diagnosis for lower backache. Because so many nerves emerge from the spine and pass through areas that

anatomy
  conditions
    therapies
      medication
        practitioner
          other

grow spurs and develop disk bulges, there is always a risk that pressure will build against one of the nerves. The problem, however, may be overdiagnosed and many backaches attributed to a pinched nerve probably have some other cause.

T   *placebo*: a treatment with no known physical value. They occupy an important place in medical history and often help speed recovery. Their effectiveness varies with the individual and the kind of disease. In backache, where the sufferer's attitude is so important, they can often steer a patient toward recovery when more "scientific" approaches fail.

P   *podiatrist*: a practitioner who specializes in problems associated with feet. Sometimes foot or leg problems lead to backache.

C   *Pott's disease*: tuberculosis of the spine. Once familiar, it is now rarely seen.

C   *prolapsed intervertebral disk*: see slipped disk.

C   *Reiter's disease*: pain in the lower back, found most often among young men and associated with an inflammation of the urinary tract and conjunctivitis (sore eyes).

P   *rheumatologist*: a medical doctor serving arthritis patients and other people with back pain.

anatomy
  conditions
    therapies
      medication
        practitioner
          | other

T   *rhizotomy*: surgery to cut a nerve root (the part that enters the spinal cord). Spinal rhizotomy, called facet rhizotomy, is not recommended.

M   *Robaxin*: a commonly prescribed muscle relaxant used by backache sufferers.

C   *sacral radiculopathy*: common phrase for low-back pain; it implies a problem with a nerve root coming out from the sacrum.

A   *sacroiliac joint*: a joint between the sacrum (see) and pelvis (see). People have two such joints, one for each side of the body.

C   *sacroiliac joint strain*: an old-fashioned diagnosis for lower-back pain. Contemporary opinion considers sacroiliac strains to be rare.

A   *sacrum*: the bone located between the hip bones. It consists of five vertebrae. At birth they are separate, but they fuse together during early childhood. It is a continuation of the vertebrae below the lumbar spine and leads to the coccyx.

C   *Scheuermann's disease*: see adolescent kyphosis.

C   *sciatica*: a common term for lower backache, especially backache that includes pain running down the leg. Pain that continues below the knee is a symptom of serious pressure on the sciatic nerve.

anatomy
| conditions
| | therapies
| | | medication
| | | | practitioner
| | | | | other

T   *sclerotherapy*: an injection used by some osteopaths designed to cause the formation of scar tissue. Sometimes it is tried as a desperate last-resort attempt to relieve chronic back pain, but it is not recommended.

C   *scoliosis*: a severe sideways distortion of the spine. It is readily treatable by surgery, which for a severe condition is very effective during childhood but extremely uncertain in adults. Milder conditions can be treated by bracing.

C   *senile kyphosis*: "hunchback," or forward curvature of the spine, caused by the loss of water in the spinal disks.

T   *Shiatsu*: a Japanese massage technique that concentrates on acupuncture points. In some cases the masseur walks on a person's back. No one with a backache should allow this part of the technique.

C   *shingles*: a viral disease that can cause backache by attacking a nerve of the lower back. It is often misdiagnosed until the appearance of a characteristic skin rash about a week after the back attack. It more often affects nerves of other parts of the body, such as the chest or face.

C   *short-leg syndrome*: mismatched leg lengths. The condition can cause backache. It is easily correctable with orthotics (see).

anatomy
  conditions
    therapies
      medication
        practitioner
          other

C   *slipped disk*: a popular diagnosis for any unexplained lower backache. Although the disk may protrude or rupture, it does not actually slip. From the 1930s into the 1970s it was routinely diagnosed for backache and often treated with surgery. Contemporary medical opinion holds that protruding and ruptured disks are relatively rare and surgery is justified only in a minority of cases.

C   *spina bifida occulta*: a birth defect in which the vertebrae are only partially formed. It does not cause back pain.

T   *spinal fusion*: a surgical attempt to correct instability in the spine by joining two or more vertebrae. It is a procedure to be approached cautiously. The back will be stiff forevermore at the point of surgery. Sometimes this effect results in extra mobility above or below the fusion and so a second operation is performed to stabilize the spine after the first fusion.

A   *spine*: the system of vertebrae that bears the load, bends with the movement, controls the motion, and protects the spinal cord of the body. Its double task of motion and support complicates its function and organization. It is divided into cervical (neck), thoracic (mid-back), lumbar (lower back), sacrum (pelvis), and coccyx (tail) regions.

anatomy
   conditions
      therapies
         medication
            practitioner
               other

A   *spinous processes*: the bony knobs on the vertebrae where muscles and ligaments attach themselves.

C   *spondylolisthesis*: the slipping forward of an individual vertebra so that it is out of line with the rest of the spine. Many athletes are at increased risk for it; these include bowlers, gymnasts, and backpackers.

C   *spondylosis*: a degeneration of the joints of the spine.

O   *Stoicism*: an approach to pain that stresses heroic bravery. Although it can be helpful in the face of short-lived acute pain, this stiff-upper-lip attitude does not work so well with chronic pain.

C   *subluxation*: a chiropractic term meaning misalignment. When medical doctors use the term they mean a partial dislocation, as in a subluxation of the shoulder.

T   *TENS* (transcutaneous electrical nerve stimulation): electric stimulation of the source of back pain. The idea is that it jams nerve signals just like some countries jam foreign radio broadcasts. It may increase body production of endorphins (see) to fight pain. It does not completely eliminate pain, but it can reduce it enough so that patients can do the exercises that will help them re-

anatomy
| conditions
| | therapies
| | | medication
| | | | practitioner
| | | | | other

        cover. The TENS machine can be worn attached to the belt while wearers go about their business.

A   *thoracic spine*: the mid-back region of the spine and the most stable part of the system. It consists of twelve vertebrae, each of which is attached to a pair of ribs. The ribs keep this part of the spine relatively immobile. It is also known as the dorsal spine. Very little back pain traces to this area.

T   *traction*: a system of pulleys and straps used to lock a patient into a still position. The original idea was to relieve pressure on the vertebrae, but research shows you need an unacceptably large force for that plan to work. Whenever it is recommended ask why bed rest will not serve just as well.

M   *Tylenol*: a common analgesic for moderate backache. The active ingredient is acetaminophen (see).

O *ultrasonography*: a tool for measuring the spinal canal's diameter by timing the echo from an ultrasonic signal.

T   *ultrasound*: a technique for producing heat below the skin by generating sound waves. Simpler techniques are thought to be just as effective, but none can provide such deep-heating relief.

anatomy
   conditions
      therapies ·
         medication
            practitioner
              other

M   *Valium*: brand name for diazepam (see).

A   *vertebra* (plural, vertebrae): a bone of the spine. In order to provide flexibility, vertebrae are relatively short bones separated by joints. They are not long bones, as in the arm or leg, where flexibility is possible only in joints at the knees and elbows. Running through the center of a vertebra is a hollow space occupied by the spinal cord. A number of knobs and cavities appear on each vertebra as points of attachment for ligaments and muscles. The ligaments hold the vertebrae in place. The muscles permit the vertebrae to move and adapt to other movements throughout the body.

M   *Vicodin*: a common analgesic for moderate to severe backache.

T   *visualization*: an important stress-reduction technique (see Chapter 1).

C   *whiplash*: popular name for chronic pain in the back of the neck.

T   *yoga*: a method of relaxation and conscious body control developed in ancient India. Its exercises are considered wonderful at keeping a healthy back in good shape, but they are risky to do during backache periods.

INDEX